The Horse Owner's Guide to
Holistic Medicine

The Horse Owner's ~Guide to~ Holistic Medicine

Sara Wyche

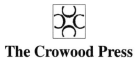

The Crowood Press

First published in 1996 by
The Crowood Press Ltd
Ramsbury, Marlborough
Wiltshire SN8 2HR

This impression 1999
© Sara Wyche 1996

British Library Cataloguing-in-Publication Data

A catalogue record for this book is available from the British Library.

ISBN 1 85223 942 5

Dedication
To Ming and Barnaby

Photographs and line-drawings by the author.

Typeset and designed by D & N Publishing, Ramsbury, Wiltshire.
Printed and bound by WBC Book Manufacturers, Bridgend, Mid Glamorgan.

ACKNOWLEDGEMENTS

Every horse is special, every horse and rider a unique combination. In some way they will all have played a part in the making of this book. Nevertheless, this book was written in Devon and it is the horses of Devon that have most recently contributed to its content.

My special thanks to the riders and horses of Ambrook Stables, Ipplepen, for allowing themselves to be photographed, and to my friend, Jim, for supporting this work with criticism, correction and best of all, encouragement.

CONTENTS

INTRODUCTION

Eye of newt, and toe of frog.
Wool of bat, and tongue of dog ...
For a charm of powerful trouble
Like a hell broth, boil and bubble.
William Shakespeare, *Macbeth*

Most owners of horses will at some time have had to call out the vet. Whether in the case of an emergency or for routine vaccinations, the veterinary surgeon represents the same system of orthodox medicine that we are familiar with when we visit the doctor. The diagnosis will be based on organ dysfunction, and the treatment will be a prescription for a mass-produced chemical compound. There is nothing wrong with that. Humans get better and so do horses.

Alternative medicine is built on entirely different concepts, namely **energy** and **individuality**. Organ dysfunction is treated as part of a whole system which has got itself out of balance, and there are no standard prescriptions, because each system is considered to be unique to the individual patient. Practitioners of alternative medicine will talk of harmonizing the flow of energy, or correcting an energy imbalance in the body. To do this, they use substances and methods which mostly defy modern scientific analysis. Nevertheless, humans get better, and so do horses.

The building blocks for health are present in us all. The difference between good health and ill health is decided largely by our emotional make-up and the pressures of our environment. That is why not everybody will catch one person's cold, even if they are all confined in one tiny room. Whatever type of medication we choose, the body has an inner vitality which is often powerful enough to promote its own healing. The purpose of alternative medicine is to strike a chord with this vitality, and help it move as freely as possible. To remove obstacles which might interrupt this flow, it makes use of the additional energy of plants and minerals, the stimulation of needles, or even the touch of the bare human hand.

Horses are very receptive to all forms of alternative medicine. Many horsemen already employ qualified professionals to carry out specific therapies. Yet few realize the extent to which they themselves influence their horse's behaviour and ultimately his well-being. The horse lives by his senses, particularly those of sight, sound and touch. The partnership with the horse is based on communication through these senses. Sight, sound and touch are also used in many alternative therapies to stimulate healing energy in a patient. If these senses already form the basis for the art of horsemanship then it is a relatively small step for the horseman to consider using them therapeutically.

The purpose of this book is to show that horsemanship and alternative medicine share many common intentions, and that different therapies can be a natural extension of the daily care and management of the horse. In fact, in wishing to understand alternative medicine, those who try to understand horses are more than half-way there.

WHAT IS IT?

Alternative medicine: is it witchcraft, black magic, a religion, or even a science? Why, in this silicon chip, laser-beam-guided world, should there be such a growing interest in remedies of a bygone age, or therapies of past civilizations? Is it nostalgia for the old apothecary's shop, or a romantic notion about gypsy-free spirit?

Orthodox medicines can be chemically identified. They are toxicologically tested, clinically proven, and licensed. The best that can be said of many alternative medicines is that they are well documented in folklore. Is it not perverse to choose, then, a remedy that has been prepared by diluting and shaking a naturally occurring substance until that substance is no longer detectable, in preference to the quality-controlled products of multi-million dollar pharmaceutical firms? Even more contrary, to stick needles the size of hatpins into points of the anatomy, along imaginary lines of energy that were conceived over 2,000 years ago! We might choose to adopt these methods for treating our own problems, but should we behave so frivolously with our horses' health?

In days gone by, horses were treated with an array of quite alarming veterinary medicines comprising heavy metals, halogens and herbs, which were combined to form blisters, embrocations, purges and drenches, in all manner of permutations for internal and external use on the horse. For example, old textbooks would list and recommend the use of such substances as aloes, arsenic, cannabis, ginger, morphine and strychnine, ointments and antiseptics using mercury, and internal 'astringents' using tincture of iron perchloride.

Nowadays, textbooks might include lists of the most modern drugs in equine practice, with their correct substance and trade name catalogued in simple alphabetical order. Chemically speaking. however, there is not much to choose between the old and the new. Modern medicines may be therapeutically more selective, and more 'user-friendly', even more palatable to the horse, but they still consist of substances that are not usually acceptable to body tissue. Acetylpromazine (ACP), or phenylbutazone (Bute) are no more a part of the body's natural metabolism, than were previously a solution of Barbados aloes or potassium iodide. The difference is that the new medicines are available only from veterinary surgeons. They are supplied only in accordance with a diagnosis made by that professional. The old remedies, crude or barbaric as they might have been, were dispensed directly to the horseman, based on his own understanding of the horse's condition.

At the time of writing, feed merchants and saddlery shops alike are giving over a vast amount of shelf space to equine health care products. The canisters and tubs may not contain morphine or strychnine, but they do claim to offer relief from such conditions as arthritis and treatments for nervousness, hormone problems and breathing problems; there are pick-me-ups for blood disorders, viral infections and even signs of old age. Home remedies may have been thrown out of the textbook, but the concept of self-help has found its way back into the horse world with a vengeance.

Similarly there are many instances where practitioners other than veterinary surgeons are being called in to treat equine health care problems. Previously it might have been just the farrier. Now the non-veterinary specializations include dentistry, behavioural problems, physiotherapy and different forms of spinal manipulation. Equine emergencies such as colics and injuries are still absolute veterinary responsibilities, and specialist equine referral clinics provide accurate and sophisticated medical diagnoses. Yet these two functions, like bookends, are being pushed further and further apart by an ever-increasing repertoire of other therapeutic possibilities.

The horse's role in society has changed. As recently as during the Second World War the horse was logistically important as a means of transport. Since then it has been superceded by the developments of science and technology. The use of the horse in competitive sport or leisure is no longer a fringe benefit of its more important function in agriculture, transport and battle. It has become its *raison d'être*. Nevertheless, when horses were a necessity, they were also more familiar. Nowadays there is a stronger tradition in car maintenance than there is in horse management!

Now, in a time of comparative economic good fortune, the horse has been reinstated – as a companion animal. However, it is no longer a horse-orientated environment. There is fierce competition for land and space, and traditional riding country is given over to other non-horse orientated leisure pursuits. Large numbers of horses are concentrated into small areas of countryside. Natural, free-roaming grazing habits are condensed into safely guarded paddocks. Social groups of horses are often dictated by necessity, rather than held together by inclination, and office hours are often responsible for unphysiological feeding practices. Many horses are ridden in unnatural or poorly balanced postures, either because of the consistency of the working surface or owing to the camber of the road. Since it is often the imbalances in the horse's environment that cause imbalance in the horse's system, and since horses and their owners have only limited resources available to them, it is not surprising that there is growing emphasis on equine health maintenance.

Absence of infection or inflammation does not automatically mean good health. Outright disease can be treated with antibiotics, anti-inflammatories and steroids, but these are specific weapons for specific wars. There are many underlying disturbances of health that can benefit from a more 'diplomatic' therapeutic approach, rather than having to withstand the immediate onslaught of heavy artillery. This is the capacity of alternative medicine.

Horse owners are now beginning to explore therapies which encourage health, rather than immediately turning to those which simply take away disease. The body has the resources to balance its own health, but if it is using a great deal of energy merely to maintain the status quo, it can surely benefit from a little extra support, especially when that health is threatened. Alternative therapies have an affinity with body tissue, or function. The techniques and substances used are all thought to have a common resonance with some part of the body's metabolism. They provide natural sources of energy, which is often potent enough to make the use of synthetic drugs unnecessary.

Alternative medicine defies scientific analysis. The evidence in support of its success is mostly anecdotal, but the results of treatment have been observed over hundreds, if not thousands, of years. Not a science, then, although some advocates might possibly want to make it a religion, but definitely no hocus-pocus. The increased availability of alternative medicine for horses has been created by the demands of the horseman. It is the result of a new awareness, a greater degree of observation, and a single-minded pursuit of what is best for the horse's health. In return, alternative medicine may enable a youthful tradition of horse management once again to come of age.

THE LANGUAGE OF HEALING

Today we say that healing is an art, but we refer to medicine as a science; language has a curious way of getting hold of the wrong end of the stick. Of course, language is only a collection of words, but the way in which we put words together reflects the way we think, and that is a product of the age we live in. The dictionary describes art as a *creative skill*, and science as *systematic and formulated knowledge*. Yet there have been times in the history of mankind when healers were thought to possess the power of scientists, and doctors (and vets) were licensed to practise the art of medicine.

Both art and science require imagination. The scientists who develop our medicine must have creative vision if they are continually to supply us with new forms of treatment. And yet, in practice, conventional medicine is often far from imaginative, using standard formulae to treat standard conditions, unable to take into account the individuality of the patient or the individual circumstances of his disease. Modern medicines are highly successful at alleviating symptoms, yet few if any of them actively encourage healing; and there *is* a difference. The conventional veterinary prescription,

'Box rest and Bute', will relieve the pain of a horse's injury and minimize the risk of further damage, but it does nothing to promote the positive rebuilding of the injured tissue.

Alternative medicine is not the result of scientific analysis in the modern sense. It has evolved out of clinical observation. Common to all forms of alternative medicine is the fact that clinicians observe what happens to the patient as an individual. The results of these observations have been recorded over thousands of years. The wealth of data which has given rise to such forms of treatment as acupuncture, homeopathy or chiropractic, is all based on clinical experience, and the sheer volume of this experience is more than a match for the comparatively short history of clinical trials in modern medicine.

Some forms of alternative medicine are centuries old, others have looked to ancient traditions for their medical philosophy. As the practitioner's skills developed into precise therapies, words had to be coined to describe the phenomena and techniques which formed the basis for treatment. Much of this terminology is old-fashioned, and the unfamiliar words are a stumbling block to modern ears. Homeopathy talks of potencies, modalities and miasms; acupuncture works through energy channels classed as Yin or Yang, along which we find Shu points, Mu points and Luo points – not only ancient, but foreign with it!

Indulging in the use of highly specialized, archaic jargon is a good way to discourage the use of any system, however worthwhile it may be. Nevertheless, jargon is a form of language, and language can be learnt. We all learn our own language long before it is formally taught to us at school. We simply practise putting words together until we provoke a meaningful response. The more we experiment, the more we develop the ability to communicate. Learning to use alternative medicine has much in common with learning a new language. The words and concepts they describe will be foreign at first, but by trying them out we gradually get a feel for their meaning.

The best way to learn about alternative medicine is to put it into practice, with ourselves, and our horses. The moment we get a positive response, we can already begin to increase the choice of therapies. The more experience we gather, the more versatile our approach to solving a problem.

There is no reason why alternative medicine should be used unscientifically, any more than the practice of scientific medicine should be unimaginative. If we can combine systematic knowledge with creative skill, we have the true language of healing.

1
LIVING ENERGY

I succeeded in discovering the cause of generation and life; nay, more, I became capable myself of bestowing animation upon lifeless matter.

Mary Shelley, *Frankenstein*

Aromatherapists do it through the nose, acupuncturists do it with needles, herbalism does it with plants, and homoeopaths can do it with minerals. The osteopath and the chiropractor both do it with bones, and the healer does it with an aura. Whatever the method, alternative medicine does it with energy!

Alternative medicine is said to be natural because it makes use of naturally occurring substances rather than synthetic products, or because it uses direct manipulative skills rather than machines. This is only partly correct; for example, the remedies of homoeopathy are certainly not in their natural state when they are applied therapeutically, and many of the tissue responses generated by different forms of manipulation can now be produced by the machines used in physiotherapy. Sticking needles into the flesh is not exactly

natural, and even less so when these are heated by setting fire to a wad of a smelly herb called Mugwort. The quality of 'naturalness' really characterizes the intention of all forms of alternative medicine to promote health by stimulating the body's own resources.

The healing of physical structures involves repair. Whether you are mending a broken bone or a broken washing machine, there are certain elementary requirements. Firstly, there are the structural ingredients: new parts or adapted old materials. Secondly, there is the act of putting the parts into the existing model. Thirdly, there is effort.

If we think of the body in its bold, anatomical structures – muscles, ligaments, bones, nerves and blood vessels, or of the inner organs – it is not hard to imagine how injury to any of these might be repaired by surgery. The ingredients for repair are provided by the sutures, a prosthesis, or a transplant organ. The operation is carried out with surgical techniques and instruments, and the effort is on the part of the surgeon. However, there are many dysfunctions of the body for which surgery would be of no use at all, yet these too need to be repaired.

The body consists of cells, which are banded together to form colonies. This is what we observe as internal organs, nerves or parts of the musculo-skeletal system. Each cell has a life of its own and is subject to individual wear and tear, and injury. The healthy body makes ample provision for a small turnover of spent cells. For example, blood cells are periodically replaced, with both the white cells which fight infection, and the red cells, which supply the body with oxygen. Worn out cells are dismantled, and their useful parts recycled into replacement cells. At this level, it is the body itself which provides the materials, the techniques *and* the effort for repair and regeneration.

In order to work, the body depends on a combination of physical forces and chemicals: physics and chemistry. The building blocks for the chemicals are chemical molecules. They give the cell walls their shape, provide the cells with food, and are the substance of cell reproduction. Molecules have always got to be on the move, otherwise life itself would come to a standstill. All molecules carry electrical charges, which enable them to be attracted to or repelled by other molecules. These electrical charges collectively produce electrical potential, which is then responsible for moving the molecules in and out of different cells. Everywhere in the body, a chemical reaction is accompanied by a change in electrical potential and followed by transport. We observe this activity as nerve signals, muscle contractions, heart beats, digestive functions and brain waves. Every process in the body is an exchange, of the physical for the chemical, and vice versa, and no such exchange can be made without producing energy.

Scientists have learnt how to keep small numbers of cells alive and working, by putting them in a glass container and feeding them an optimum diet. Obviously cells in the body do not live in this sort of splendid isolation. There are external influences, competition for nourishment, and dependence on the efficiency of neighbouring cells. Cell functions not only create energy, they use it; and it is the energy resource which, at times, may be quite thinly spread to satisfy the minimum requirements of all concerned. If the energy becomes depleted then one part of the body may find itself in real trouble. This energy deficit will sooner or later make itself outwardly apparent as a collection of symptoms which we identify as illness.

Our modern system of medicines is based on chemistry, not physics, and does not take into account the state of energy imbalance which must occur when a body is unwell. In fact, modern medicine often gives the body more work to do, since all the substances have to be metabolized and eliminated, both of which are energy-intensive processes.

Modern medicines fall into the following broad categories:
• Those that combat infection.
• Those that calm inflammation.
• Those that correct hormones.
• Those that modify chemical mediators.
The concept behind most of our modern drugs is one of conquering, suppressing, supplanting, controlling; as if the body

was just an empty landscape upon which to create a battlefield. The *Medical Speciality Index* reads like a list of 'antis': antibacterials, antifungals, antivirals, antipyretics, antipruritics, antiemetics, antidepressants. Modern pharmacology is the science of being 'against': we might be prescribed something *for* a cough, or *for* a headache, but what we receive is actually against the cough and against the headache, and certainly not *for* the chest, or *for* the head.

That is not to say that modern medicines should never have been invented, or that their use is not justified in treating illness. The world would not, of course, be a better place without penicillin, vaccines, or chemotherapy. There are many situations where the amount of energy required by the body, either to regain health by manufacturing its own substances, or even just to 'hold the fort', is so considerable that to send in an army of chemicals is the only option. The advantages of dispatching a biological invader as quickly and thoroughly as possible more than outweighs the possible disadvantages (i.e. side-effects). Yet, after any battle there is always the task of clearing up, repairing and rebuilding, and this applies just as much to the body in the aftermath of disease.

For example, antibiotics can kill infection by inhibiting the growth or reproduction of bacteria. The presence of bacteria is, nevertheless, also recognized by substances in the body's bloodstream. These substances pass on the information to the white blood cells, and a well-rehearsed strategy for dealing with invaders is put into operation. By the time the antibiotics arrive a little war is already in progress. As the germs are destroyed there is a build-up of debris from the dead bacteria and the dead blood cells. The antibiotics are also spent, like any ammunition, and they too have to be removed. This period of tidying up requires energy, but apart from some vitamin tonics there are no modern pharmaceuticals that can assist this return to wellness, as opposed to those that were prescribed to deal with the illness. Yet recovering from illness can be more demanding on the body's energy than the conquest itself.

Similarly, the symptoms of inflammation – redness, swelling, heat, and possibly itching or pain – are part of a complex chain of responses, involving cells, cell messengers, and mediator substances. Inflammation is the body's response to, for example, excess pressure or compression, the presence of an irritant, or even the body at odds with itself. The symptoms are part of the healing strategy: heat and redness are signs of increased circulation, which enables the materials for repair to be transported into the area and damaged elements to be removed. Even the pain has a purpose, serving both as a distress signal and as a focus for the repair forces.

Corticosteroids are often prescribed to relieve inflammation. Yet the body produces its own 'steroids' in response to many different kinds of stimuli. The important point is that the body also produces other substances which control the steroid level. This regulatory system is more finely tuned than anything that can be administered in the form of medication. This is why steroid therapy brings with it the risk of side-effects.

Anti-inflammatories of the non-steroidal type, like aspirin or (in horses) Bute, are almost *too* effective in their pain-relieving and anti-inflammatory effects: they are so successful that the body is no longer aware that it has a problem. It takes no more steps towards active healing because the problem has, apparently, ceased to exist.

Most modern medicines represent scientific triumphs in problem-solving. There are drugs that can fit like keys into the molecular structure of the body. Yet, however brilliantly these substances can slot into a biological process, they never actually become part of it. The body does not suddenly begin synthesizing drugs like beta blockers or bronchodilators, just because they are doing a grand job. Modern medicines help to manage illness; they don't necessarily give us health.

REACHING THE SOURCE OF ILLNESS

To achieve their full therapeutic effect, modern pharmaceuticals have to reach a certain concentration at the site where they are actually needed. To do this they all use a common route, the bloodstream. It's an obvious choice, since all the major ports of entry into the body are well served by a dense network of blood vessels, close to the surface. The blood circulation ensures that what starts at one end will be taken to every corner of the body, providing there is enough to go round.

The make-up of the blood is very carefully controlled. Solid and fluid components have to be finely regulated so that the blood does not become too viscous and particles do not interfere with each other's function. Therapeutic substances have to abide by the same parameters. Blood vessels vary greatly in size, from the dimensions of the major arteries down to the miniscule capillaries, where it is a tight squeeze for even one red blood cell to get through. The bloodstream might be a popular means of transport, but when it's overloaded with medication it resembles something between the London Underground at rush hour and an old sewer.

The bloodstream is a favourite means of 'public transport' for modern medicines because its system has been mapped out in the greatest detail, from the major trunk road to the smallest lane, and even the pathways leading to the door of every cell. Yet like any communication network, the bloodstream is not infallible. In areas where the body is suffering from disease or dysfunction, the blood circulation is generally not in perfect working order. Using this route as a means of providing medication is equivalent to trying to reach the scene of a road accident by ambulance, when the roads are blocked by traffic. It is not always the most efficient way to provide help.

Not all forms of medicine rely for their delivery on transport via the bloodstream. Imagine you are sitting in your car on a four-lane motorway – in a traffic jam. It might be a comfortable car, even a technologically advanced car, but it isn't going anywhere. Ahead, there are several bridges visible, all providing for different modes of transport: there are railway lines, waterways, even walkways. Then, above those, there are air-

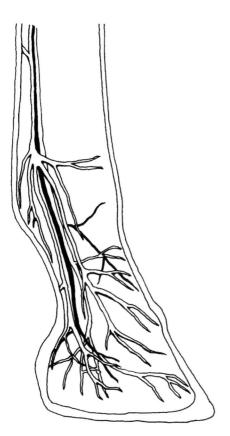

Even just below the skin of the horse's forelimb an extensive system of nerves more than parallels the arterio-venous supply.

channels, small blood vessels with few particles, large blood vessels chock-a-block, muscle fibres, tendons, ligaments, and bones. These are *all* communication systems. They can all, potentially, be 'spoken to'. The body itself does not always respond to a problem by taking the circuitous route of the bloodstream. Nerves, for example, are enormously useful structures. They are constructed like telephone wires with junction boxes, and their fibres extend the length and breadth of the body. They are capable of passing information in milliseconds. Getting on the right side of the nervous system can really get things done around the body. We can influence nerves so that they do not transmit pain messages, we can encourage them to move muscles. We can induce them to produce transmitter substances, which themselves are powerful healers. Information from the nerves will stimulate the production of these.

Apart from nerves, there is communication by water. The body is fairly swimming in it. If we throw a stone into a pond, it causes ripples that spread in every direction. There are alternative therapies which are thought to apply their energy to the body in a similar way.

The body makes use of electricity in its life functions. Unless every structure were carefully insulated from its neighbour, there must be an overlapping and interaction of all the electricity energy fields. Patterns of electrical energy lines are formed, which in the healthy body travel along constant pathways. If an area of the body becomes ill, the flow of energy will be interrupted and the pattern will change. Western medicine has not tried to map *these* pathways, and so

craft, as well as any number of telephone wires and other communication cables. Now imagine you are a microscopic entity taking a journey through a cross-section of the body, perhaps a finger or a forelimb. After passing through the outermost layer of the skin, you will encounter the following structures: sensor cells in different shapes, nerve fibres in all sorts of thicknesses, watery fluid, some of it in defined makes no use of them therapeutically. Nevertheless, other cultures have observed these phenomena, and made detailed records of the existence of energy channels. To us they might be as invisible as the Equator or the North Pole, but that does not mean to say they are not there.

Life cannot exist without energy, and neither can healing. The chemical and physical properties of the body can be measured, and these are evidence enough of the existence of a living energy. Yet nobody has been able to define its exact nature. That would probably amount to discovering the secret of 'Eternal Life', and no form of medicine pretends that it has done that. Nevertheless, we may all acknowledge that there is a natural force in every living being, and that this natural force has the power to heal. Harnessing this potential is the most essential requirement of all alternative medicine.

2
CHOOSING AN ALTERNATIVE

'Well, I'll eat it', said Alice, 'and if it makes me grow larger, I can reach the key; and if it makes me grow smaller, I can creep under the door: so either way I'll get into the garden.'

Lewis Carroll, *Alice's Adventures in Wonderland*

THE RAW MATERIAL

Food is a commodity – a raw material – that comes in so many guises that without some form of categorization we would be unable to choose the items required for building a balanced diet. However, the categories can be created to satisfy different specifications. For example, supermarkets arrange our food in line with our eating *habits* (vegetables, meat, bread); nutritionists classify our food according to *needs* (protein, carbohydrates and fat). We can choose between beef and pork, because these are two kinds of meat, but we can also choose between protein and fat by selecting a lean cut as opposed to a fatty one. To go shopping we need some knowledge of the one system; to come home with a sensible diet, we need some understanding of the other system.

Like food, alternative medicine is a commodity. Its raw material is energy. Energy is not so easy to visualize as the constituents of food, like protein or carbohydrates. Nevertheless, we have plenty of evidence of its existence. Atomic energy, thermal energy, electromagnetic energy; we see it in the natural world, we manufacture it to provide our homes with creature comforts, and if we so much as lift a finger, well, we've used it to do that as well.

Energy, therefore, is not something we should single out as an entity separate from ourselves. It is all around us and within us. Our senses constantly monitor it in all its forms. We see light, we hear vibrations, we feel the tingling of heat or cold. This enables our biological energy to keep pace with our environment. It is a constant balancing act, and even the best balancing acts in the world have been known to wobble. Rebalancing the energy is the purpose of alternative medicine.

Almost anything that affects our senses, makes our hearts beat faster or lifts our spirits, can rightfully be called alternative medicine. Sunlight makes us cheerful, the greenness of woods and fields is soothing to the eyes, and the tinkling of a stream can unwind busy minds. Feeling a warm sandy beach under bare feet is the beginning of reflexology, pebbly shingle even more so. Dangling your legs in running water is a form of hydrotherapy, rubbing the elbow of a child who has fallen over, the first step in acupressure, and a hot cup of tea is a herbal infusion. Alternative therapies have grown up from the observation of simple phenomena, the effect of smell, the touch of a hand, the buoyancy of water. Yet they are now all wrapped up as such individual packages that it is hard to remember that they are simply different approaches to the practice of energy medicine.

SELECTING A THERAPY

Selecting the most appropriate treatment, particularly for animal therapy, is like standing in front of the home-bakery stall at a village fête: should we take home a jar of homoeopathy, or an acupuncture cake, a pie filled with fresh physiotherapy, or a chiropractic preserve? Each therapy lures us with its tantalizing mixture of individuality and age-old tradition, and the choice we make might be as random as choosing strawberry jam

rather than chocolate cake. Alternative medicine is not usually presented in a way that allows us to make comparative or selective judgements.

Just as it is possible to *decide* how much protein to eat, *choose* the sort of quality it should have, and *elect* to combine it with a little or even a lot of fat, so we should be able to base our selection of natural therapy on the requirements and relevance of what we want to treat, rather than on limited availability or popular hearsay. At first glance it might seem impossible to make such a deliberate choice when there appears to be no overall system of organization for the many types of alternative therapies. Is it feasible to impose such a system on therapies as diverse as osteopathy, aromatherapy and radionics?

Any systematic arrangement of alternative therapies will not be able to take into account *all* the nuances and idiosyncrasies of the different approaches. Yet it is indeed possible to organize alternative medicine into themes, based on the different methods of treatment. The system of categorization below came about when it was observed that the stimulus to promote natural healing can be applied at different levels.

Groups of therapies share common characteristics in the way they stimulate healing. Some work on our outer senses, some manipulate us physically and some come into contact with the body's internal energy patterns. If we compare the body to a planet, energy applied to the planet's crust will be of a different dimension from that released from the planet's own core. Although it would be wrong to make judgements about the quality of healing achieved by any one form of therapy, it is true that the stimulus may be anything from a therapeutic megaphone to the tiniest whisper. Those therapies that make the least 'noise' are usually the most potent.

According to a comparison of the methods used, alternative medicine can be divided into three main categories:

1. stimulation of the senses;
2. manipulation of the musculo-skeletal system;
3. application of direct energy.

All alternative therapies can be allocated to one of these groups, though this does not make any statement about the strength or effectiveness of the individual therapies.

The system simply shows that there is progressive development in natural healing methods. They begin by using external stimuli that work via one of the five senses; the sense of touch leads logically to the skill of manipulation and the manual release of energy blocks leads to the concept of manipulating energy by more subtle means, in the form of specific energy carriers.

The list of therapies in the diagram is intentionally comprehensive. It does include therapies normally associated with human treatment – colour therapy, music therapy, reflexology – which might beg the question, should the horse-owner repaint the walls of his stable, serenade his horse, and massage the soles of the hoof? The horse world is, after all, full of colour,

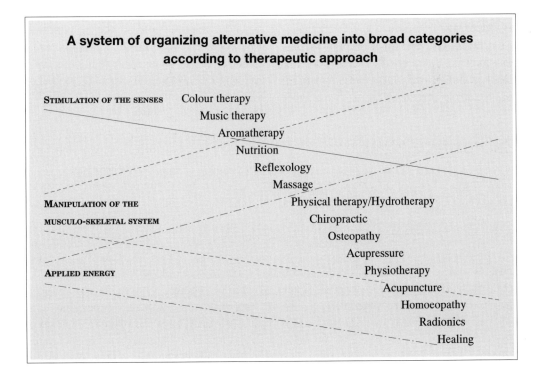

A system of organizing alternative medicine into broad categories according to therapeutic approach

STIMULATION OF THE SENSES

Colour therapy
Music therapy
Aromatherapy
Nutrition
Reflexology
Massage

MANIPULATION OF THE
MUSCULO-SKELETAL SYSTEM

Physical therapy/Hydrotherapy
Chiropractic
Osteopathy
Acupressure

APPLIED ENERGY

Physiotherapy
Acupuncture
Homoeopathy
Radionics
Healing

and horses probably see colour as well as we do. Whose horse doesn't like big red buses, or large, white, plastic-wrapped silage bales, or coloured fillers in show jumps? Why do we wear red to go hunting but not for the dressage test? Why do we pop a novice horse over a log in the woods, but take care in the way we introduce the same horse to coloured poles? This is part of the horse's education, but there is no reason to suppose that there are not health implications, too, in the use of certain colours around some horses.

Many riders will have experienced the enhanced effect that riding to music has on the horse's movements. Surely, strides carried out in a constant rhythm are more beneficial to joints and muscles than movements produced under tension. Music can give useful support in achieving fluent stride sequences.

Even though areas of the horse's body have not yet been mapped out into the soles of his feet, what else is the farrier, if not an equine reflexologist? It is *his* craft

that is in constant contact with the horse's foot. Both the shoes and the nails exert pressure, and if this is incorrect or excessive, the balance of the whole limb will change. If the movement of the limb is altered, this will cause cramps elsewhere in the body, which, eventually, will effect the space available to internal organs. Conversely, good shoeing must have a beneficial effect on the horse's health. It is not natural for horses to wear shoes so, whatever else it does, shoeing should contribute to maintaining balanced health.

With the very simplest means at our disposal, we horse owners and riders should recognize that, in the first instance, we are all practitioners of alternative medicine, just by caring for our horses. Our stable management, our pasture care, grooming and very definitely riding: this is where it all begins. If we understand how our input affects the horse in wellness then it will be possible to make a logical choice of therapy when treating the horse in illness.

3
APPEALING TO THE SENSES

'The first place that I can well remember was a large, pleasant meadow with a pond of clear water in it. Some shady trees leaned over it, and rushes and water-lilies grew at the deep end.'

Anna Sewell, *Black Beauty*

It is rather a pity that with all the film and television versions of this famous novel, we have probably all forgotten, or have never even read, these opening words of Black Beauty's story. Of course, it is a human's attempt to describe the world as it is seen by a horse, to give the impression of an idyllic backdrop for the innocent life of the young foal; a sort of equine Garden of Eden.

Would a horse really appreciate a lily pond? Wouldn't the flies be just awful, and all the horses get mud fever in the winter? This picturesque portrayal may seem a little quaint to us now, but in one respect it is entirely accurate: it puts the world of the horse firmly in the domain of the senses.

Imagine the sparkling taste of clean water, listen to the trembling of the rushes,

feel the contrasting texture of the leathery lily leaves and their silky flowers, and let your eyes rest in the dappled shade of the trees: the horse experiences the world through his senses. He is in constant contact with his environment. His senses are always on open channel, never on hold. His responses are immediate, not reflective. In the wild this was his means of survival, and just because we put him in a stable and feed him three square meals a day, does not mean that he will simply put this part of his being to one side. In fact, in our efforts to provide for and protect our horses, we are often in danger of causing considerable mental conflict. Box-walking and weaving are both habits that result from man imposing restrictive behaviour patterns onto an otherwise free spirit.

Of all the animals with which man forms a close association, the sense organs of the horse have the most distinctive features. Dogs and cats speak to us with their eyes, give us warnings with the position of

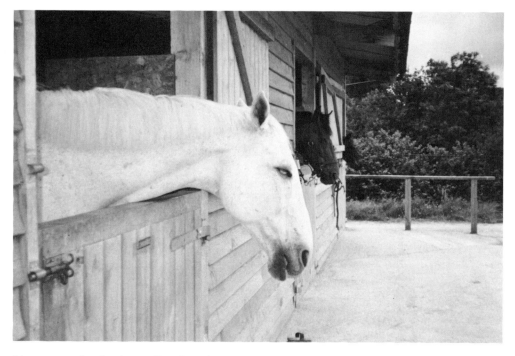

Horses need quiet times: Sunday afternoon at Ambrook Stables.

their ears, and reinforce their intentions with their voices and body language. The horse can add to all these signals with the flare of his nostrils and the shaping of his lips and muzzle. In the horse, the facial features are more demonstrative in total than in other companion animals, because they occupy more space relative to the size of the head.

It is possible that we value the company of the horse, not only because he allows us to partner him in his range of movements, but because he seems to be in such direct contact with the world. Man's evolution has been in the development of intellect: it is the ability to think, to reflect, to solve problems that sets man apart from other animals. A human being does not often need to react in an instant to a sound, a smell or a sight. He makes judgements based on information and experience. On the other hand, we almost expect the horse to react spontaneously. We then set about trying to educate him towards accepting our informed approach. Fortunately, he never abandons his own real perception of the world. If he did, he would become nothing more than a machine. He simply learns to incorporate the decisions of his rider, or handler, because he trusts them.

Unfortunately, there is also room for misunderstandings. It is not too difficult for the horse to learn the rules of the master, providing the tasks are fair and within his

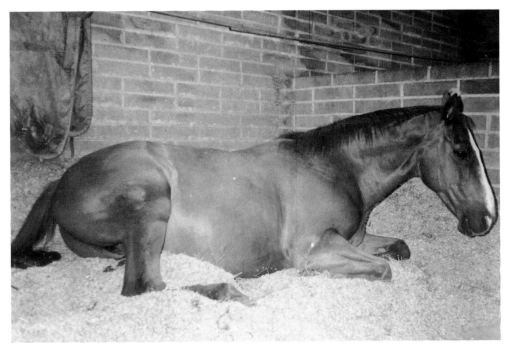

A moment to be private in a light, well-ventilated stable.

capability. It is much harder for the master to enter into the sensitivity of the horse; we would have to put aside our intellect to do so. We have to remember that we, too, are part of the horse's outside world; our gestures, our voices, our body language have a tremendous impact on his senses. He, after all, has to decide whether a swift motion of the hand is going to give him a pat, a quick flick over with a brush, or an angry reprimand. We yell at him in encouragement, we shout at him for disobedience, and we expect him to come when we bellow cross the field. We cannot possibly estimate the acuteness of the horse's senses because ours do not react with the same immediacy.

Be that as it may, human health has been positively influenced by therapies that make special use of the senses. There is no reason why we should not adapt the basic intentions of these therapies in our day-to-day horse care. Their harmonizing and restorative qualities will put us more in touch with the horse, the earth, and possibly even ourselves.

LIGHT

Being witness to the exact moment of blindness in a horse is a heart-rending experience. A mare who belonged to a veterinary colleague suffered from

Asking Questions

A consultation in any form of human alternative medicine is a lengthy process because many questions must be asked about the individual. To apply the same approach to the horse, we need to ask questions of the horse as an individual – and understand the answers. To do this, we must study the way the horse expresses itself through the five senses, and consider how these senses might be used in therapy.

periodic opthalmia. This disease often begins with quite trivial signs of an irritation at the corner of the eye but, probably due to an immune-mediated reaction, can result in massive changes within the eye itself. This mare was known to have had bouts of the disease, but only in one of her eyes. It was thought that even though there were some remnants of the process here, she probably could see just a little. Despite all precautions, however, the other eye suddenly showed signs of deterioration. It was a helpless pair of vets who looked on as the front chamber gradually filled with thick white pus, undeterred by both orthodox and alternative medicine. It then became apparent that the mare had no vision in the already diseased eye. In the space of a moment the horse became totally blind. Despite all human comforting and encouragement the mare would only stagger around, a few feet at a time. She was quite obviously terrified. It was thought that given even the slightest chance of a remission, the

distress could not be justified, and the horse was put down.

The Horse's Sight

When we look at any horse, we are first drawn to his eyes. We imagine we can interpret their expression, though we possibly see in them a reflection of our own emotions. Nevertheless, it's the eye that makes the horse an individual. From the horse's point of view, the eye is not so much a window of the soul, but more of a watch tower, permanently 'manned' to keep him in touch with his surroundings. He is not very good at focusing on objects that are directly ahead of him when these are at close range, but the position of the eyes in the skull means that he can see extremely well to either side, thus affording him a panoramic view of the world. After all, he has got to be able to gallop full speed across rough country, without tripping up and without bumping into other members of the herd. In fact the horse's vision is quite remarkable when we consider that, for example, when working on the lunge over cavaletti he can see not only the poles, but also the smallest gesture of the lunge whip, *and* keep an eye on his handler in the middle: and that's not taking into account what he's seeing on the other side.

That is not to say that horses cannot get used to having little or no sight if the loss of vision has happened very gradually. A circus horse was admitted to a veterinary clinic with an injury very close to one eye, which was the result of a kick. Only then was it discovered that he was actually

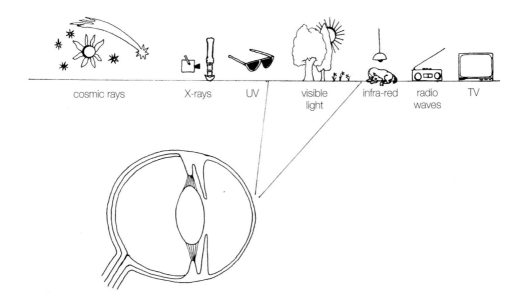

cosmic rays   X-rays   UV   visible light   infra-red   radio waves   TV

The eye receives information from only a small part of the electromagnetic spectrum.

totally blind in both eyes, and probably had been for a long time. He had been able to perform because of the nature of the routine, until, that is, he got just a bit too close to the horse in front.

Our own Trakehner mare, Oliva, had probably lived in a world of grey shadows for a couple of years. A severe virus infection around the throat and lymph glands caused an unusual immune reaction which spread to the tissues of the eye. It was only when she misjudged the branches of an overhanging tree that we realized that she couldn't see very much at all. In spite of the blindness she used to gallop across the paddock, put the brakes on near the entrance, step very cautiously through the opening, and off she'd go again at a gallop. When her foal was born, she used him as a 'guide dog', though the day eventually came when the foal lost interest in its mother, and the mare was left helplessly stranded.

Expression

The eyes of the horse, therefore, are its most important receivers of information. How much information they give out, as to the mental and emotional state of the horse, is less easy to define. Like most animals, horses make their intentions clear by changing the overall outline of the head, which involves changing the position of the ears. This, along with body posturing, is easily recognizable from a distance. It would otherwise be highly dangerous if you had to get close enough to see a change of emotion in the narrowing of the eyelids, only to find you were about to receive both barrels!

Although we cannot be certain that the eye of the horse expresses the fluctuations of emotion (as we humans understand them), one thing they definitely do express is a capacity for life. For example, a horse in the final stages of an irreversible colic no longer looks at the outside world. His eyes are not thrown open in panic, as they are in the acute onset of laminitis. The impression is that he turns his attention completely inwards, towards the very centre of his pain, and himself.

As portrait painters know, the eyes are brought to life by adding a little highlight, suggesting the reflection of light on the moist surface of the living conjunctiva. If this is missing the eyes do not hold our attention; they appear dull and expressionless. Horses' eyes become expressionless when they have experienced mental or physical trauma.

In the autumn of 1987, the south of England was the scene of an unnaturally severe storm. Most of the casualties of the 'hurricane' were trees and buildings. In a small yard near Epsom, trees did come down but the stables were new and brick-built, and suffered no structural damage. In this yard there was a most attractive,

sparky, bright bay gelding that had done well in the show ring. After the hurricane, it was noticed that his eyes had lost their highlights. He didn't stop eating, and all blood tests and organ checks showed no pathological changes; he just became lethargic and disinterested, and his eyes gave the impression that there was nobody home. The only conclusion was that the sound of the 100mph. winds passing through the high, open roof-space of the stables had caused the horse to have a nervous breakdown. It took about eighteen months for him to return to normal.

Mental distress can also lead to a horse shutting down just part of his personality. A driving team of two Polish horses was imported to the UK. They were then separated. The most interesting feature about one of the horses was his eyes, His left eye was open and trusting, whereas the right eye, though physiologically the same size, was always narrowed and suspicious-looking, In addition to this, the moment he left the stable yard he started to walk with a limp, dropping the left hip. The other horse was his brother, who had been sold on. He quickly earned the reputation of being dangerous, because twenty yards from home he would send all potential purchasers into orbit. He had never been taught to walk out by himself. He considered himself only part of a whole unit, and his 'nap' was an expression of distress. One winter's day, however, out on a hack with a substitute 'brother' on foot, he caught sight of the skyline of Dartmoor. The brightness of the winter blue sky and the sharpness of the sunshine made the colours of the moor so brilliant, they seemed close enough to touch. After that day the right eye opened, the two halves of his facial expression became symmetrical, and the hind-limb lameness completely disappeared.

Light and Colour

Light enters the eye, and is focused by the cornea and the lens so that it accurately strikes the nerve cells embedded in the back wall of the eyeball, the area called the retina. The cells respond to light stimulus by producing electrical impulses, which are transmitted along the optic nerve to the brain. The brain processes the information, and this process is what we know as 'seeing'.

Light is a form of energy, electromagnetic energy. Visible light is only the tiniest part of the whole electromagnetic spectrum of energy, which fills the entire universe. The nerve cells of the retina are adapted to the stimulus of this energy within a very narrow band of wavelengths which is approximately in the middle of the whole spectrum. Shorter wavelengths with much higher energy, such as X-ray or cosmic rays, would be harmful, and longer wavelengths, which vibrate relatively slowly, are experienced as sound.

There are two types of light-sensitive cell in the retina, rods and cones. The rods are responsible for making sense out of different light intensities and are important in night vision. The cones respond to specific wavelengths within the visible light spectrum, and these are ordered by the brain into what we consciously call colours. The retina of the horse contains more rods than that of humans, and they are thought to have better night vision than us. Anyone out hacking late will have been grateful for this! Horses are also considered to have almost as many cones as humans. Since these contain a similar range of pigments it is suggested that horses do indeed have some form of

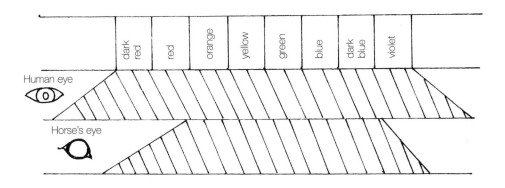

The horse's eye probably has a narrower band of colour sensitivity than the human eye.

colour vision. Interpretation of colour varies greatly among human individuals, so it is difficult to evaluate what sort of colour sense the horse has.

Work by Professor Grzimek seems to demonstrate that horses are able to distinguish between the different wavelengths that correspond to our colours yellow, green, red and blue. Colours are produced by the reflection of some wavelengths and absorption of others. For example, a blue object absorbs all the component colours of light shining on it, except blue, which it reflects. The names of colours are simply a convenient way of communicating a like sensation among humans. It is likely that the horse receives similar information since his retina is equipped to do so, and that he is affected in the same way by the different wavelengths, even though he cannot put a name to them.

Colour psychology is an established science. The colours that surround us are now chosen with special purpose, from the cars we drive, to the paint on our walls, and the packaging of our food. Manufacturers leave nothing to chance, because colour affects our state of mind. For example, the colour red keeps us alert and enhances activity, but too much red can bring out aggression. Yellow encourages detachment and shallow breathing, while green creates balance but also arrests movement. Green can help people tolerate a noisy working environment, but too much green makes them over-relaxed. Blue combats tension, and creates a feeling of breathing out, of relaxation. Blue has the energy of peace.

There would be no need to give the colour perception of the horse any more consideration if we did not try to keep him and work with him in a man-made world. A large livery yard which has to make the most use of the space available, puts up a stable block with internal loose boxes facing a central gangway; this

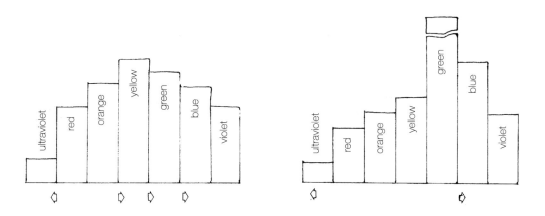

The distribution of colours in natural light compared to the distribution in fluorescent lighting.

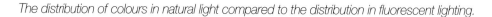

Coloured Jump Poles

The visual impact of colours in the showjumping course is largely the product of experience and tradition, rather than psychology. However, the use of colour can make a difference between a fair and an unfair test of the horse's accuracy. It is known that horses cannot see jumps clearly when they are placed against a background of the same colour. Certain colours, such as dark green, appear receding, so they should not be used at the base of a jump.

Unfortunate colour combinations can draw the horse's eye away from the poles to the wings, and plain coloured fences are more difficult to jump, than those where the surface is broken up by contrasting shapes. Shape tends to accentuate colour, and this plays a part in educating young horses. There are not many examples of large vertical, coloured surfaces on the horse's native plains, so the horse has to learn that a big red bus or lorry is an acceptable part of his adopted world.

arrangement requires artificial lighting, usually in the form of fluorescent tubes. The spectrum of light that these give out is not the same as that produced by full daylight: there is more blue and green than red. In humans, red light increases muscular activity, blood pressure and heart rate, while blue has the opposite effect. If nature provided the eye with the means to detect both colours, then it probably had a very good reason for doing so: to keep both effects in balance.

People who spend a great deal of time in artificial light, or who lack sunlight in the winter, can suffer from a real deficiency of natural light known as Seasonal Affective Disorder, or S.A.D. There are horses that spend up to twenty-three hours a day without natural light; if they work in an indoor school as well, then twenty-four!

There are two other mechanisms in the eye, which have been the subject of investigation in the horse. One is the abil-ity to focus, and the other is the length of time it takes for the eye to adapt to sudden changes of light. The evidence found from examination of the anatomical structures suggests that the horse probably doesn't focus well at close range, and that his eyes take much longer to adjust to a change of light than ours do. In fact, sudden changes may even be quite uncomfortable.

On the basis that 'a rest is as good as a cure', a sick horse is often prescribed a period of box rest for several weeks or even months. He then spends this time in an enclosed space, where everything is not quite in focus, bathed in an artificial light that has an unbalanced colour spectrum – and he's supposed to get better?

Light as a Treatment

There is literally more to light than meets the eye! The eye is sensitive to the wavelengths of visible light, but the body as a whole is sensitive to wavelengths on either side of the colour spectrum, namely ultra-violet and infra-red. Ultra-violet light contains wavelengths that are potentially harmful, and for this reason has fallen into disrepute. We tend to forget that ultra-violet light is responsible for many important photochemical and photobiological processes in the body, of which vitamin D synthesis is the most well known.

Respiratory infections caused by viruses are now widespread among the horse population. The more serious ones are prevented by vaccination programmes, but others can be debilitating enough and put horses out of action for quite some time. It is not unusual for blood tests, taken long after the actual infection has passed, to show that the red and white blood-cell populations have not quite made it back to their normal status. It may only be a minimal deficit, but the horses are just 'one degree under'. It is not pure speculation to suggest that the availability of sunlight might have something to do with this problem.

A German manufacturer of equine solaria commissioned a study into the effects of solarium use in horses that were stabled for long periods of time. The type of solarium used produced UV-A, visible, and infra-red light, and the horses were given fifteen minutes' treatment daily, about half the normally recommended treatment time. All the horses showed signs of deep relaxation under the lamps, one foal even lay flat out on its side next to its mother. Blood samples were taken to monitor the effects on the red blood cells.

It was found that the number of red blood cells steadily increased, as did the haemoglobin. The leucocyte/lymphocyte ratio, which often changes during infection, quickly changed in favour of the normal healthy white cell distribution. There was also an improvement in heart, pulse, and respiratory rate recovery times after exercise, indicating a positive effect of the light therapy on the nerves which regulate these functions.

A solarium probably sounds like an expensive luxury to most horse owners. However, if owners from half a dozen livery yards were to add up the amount of money they spent on the coughing horse, in the form of veterinary fees and medication, antibiotics, bronchodilators, mucolytics and garlic, not to mention loss of riding hours, they would probably find that a regular dose of artificial sunshine was actually an affordable alternative.

In humans, the use of coloured light to treat physical and emotional disorders is a complex therapy involving not only the knowledge of colour psychology but also the ability to tune into the energy imbalances along the spine and into the layers of energy which surround the physical body. There is no reason why this should not be applied to the horse. There are people who have developed their ability to see these energy layers, called auras, and who can sense the fluctuations of energy in them. Such people have a beneficial effect on those they treat. However, it is not really necessary for us to go looking for concepts in the realms of spiritual philosophy; all *we* have to do is open our eyes to the horse.

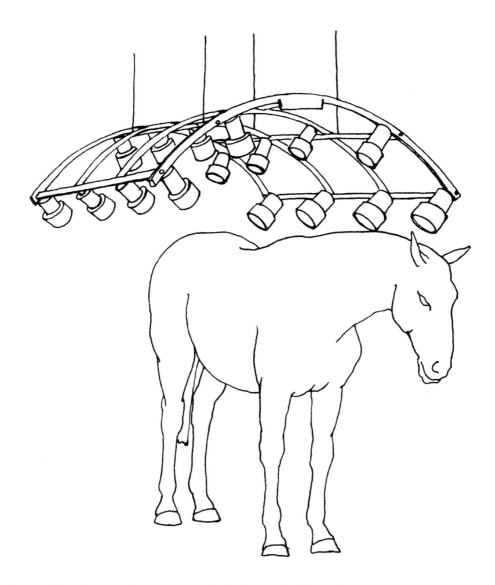

The solarium has many health benefits for the horse, including relaxation.

Light Summary

1. Eyesight is probably the most important of the five senses to the horse.
2. Energy, in the form of light, is received by the retina and passed on as electrical impulses to the visual cortex of the brain.
3. Some of this information is received by an area of the brain called the hypothalamus, which in turn influences the pituitary and pineal glands. These glands regulate the body's biological clock, and the production of adrenal and sexual hormones, according to the type of light received.
4. The horse can distinguish between different wavelengths of the visible light spectrum, which we describe as colours.
5. Shape gives more definition to colour. Combinations of shape and colour can prove a fair or unfair test of a horse's ability.
6. Humans make an intuitive choice of colour in their dress and their surroundings. The colours we choose reflect our physical and emotional states. The horse is sensitive to these emotions, such as calmness, excitement, tension, anger. Understanding our colour preference can help us be more objective about our influence on the horse.
7. The horse's eye expresses his own physical and mental well-being.
8. For the short, rain-filled days of autumn and winter, as a prophylaxis or pick-me-up, artificial sunlight may be a worthwhile alternative. In many sophisticated, ancient civilizations, sunlight was the ultimate form of healing-energy medicine.

SOUND

The Ear

Sound is a form of energy, caused by vibration. The ear translates this sensory information into electrical impulses. Incoming sound waves are focused by the outer ear canal onto the ear-drum, or tympanic membrane. This vibrates in sympathy and, via three individually shaped, tiny bones, causes the next membrane to do the same. Behind this is a snail-shaped compartment, which contains a liquid. There are thousands of minute hair-like fibres suspended in this liquid, which are bent as the vibrations pass along it. This deformation triggers an electrical impulse, which travels along the auditory nerve to the brain.

If we think about all the sounds that we can recognize, apparently simultaneously, it is remarkable that these are first of all received by a rather undistinguished flap of skin, which makes up the ear-drum. In humans this membrane is about 0.25in (6mm) in diameter. Yet a concert-goer can listen to a hundred-piece symphony orchestra, distinguish individual instruments, take in the accompaniment of a choir of voices, hear someone cough in the next row and register a bus pulling up outside. In the horse, anatomists have estimated the ear-drum to be smaller than that of humans; it is approximately 0.2mm thick. We can only speculate whether this makes a horse's ear-drum more or less sensitive than ours.

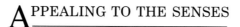

Human beings do not carry ear trumpets unless they are deaf. The horse, however, has his ear trumpets permanently attached to the sides of his head, and these are manipulated by twenty-two tiny muscles. We can get an impression of what this is like if we cup our hand around an ear lobe. It enables us to pick up an individual sound more precisely against a background of noise.

The Effect of Sound on the Heart-Rate

To understand how sound affects the heart-rate, we must look at the function of muscles and the purpose of the nervous system. There are three types of muscle in the body: smooth muscle cells, which form the walls of the inner organs; skeletal muscle cells, which are part of the locomotor system; and heart muscle cells, which have the combined characteristics of both the other two types. All types of muscle cell have the potential for spontaneous contraction, so they all have to underlie some higher system of organization. Regulating the exact order in which muscular contractions occur is the function of the nervous system. The nerves that instruct the skeletal system operate separately from those that co-ordinate the contractions of inner organs, for obvious reasons. We might not want to be concerned with the inch by inch passage of our food along the intestine, but in the event of a tummy upset we might want to instruct our limbs to get us as quickly as possible to the nearest W.C. It would also be inconvenient if our hearts stopped beating every time we forgot to think about

them. Therefore the nervous system is divided into two categories: voluntary for locomotion and involuntary for internal functions.

The two systems are independently regulated, but they do have their point of origin in the same brain. There are crossover points in the brain, and in other parts of the body. Information can be passed between the two systems by transmitter substances and hormones. The voluntary and involuntary nerves have to keep each other informed, so that the whole body can respond as a unit. If a body suddenly has to run for its life, it needs muscle power, fuel and a fully active fuel pump. An idling heart beat, and sluggish blood circulation are not much use to muscles that have to leap into action. Sound is one stimulus: it may cause increased activity in the voluntary nerves, and it may also unconsciously stimulate the involuntary ones,

Solitaire was a 16.2hh., eleven-year-old, Irish-bred gelding. He was examined for purchase on a rather warm, lazy afternoon at a small professional, show-jumping yard. He was handsomely put together, an eventing-type Thoroughbred, with good substance and bone, well-defined joints, and an obedient, laid-back disposition. He completed all the stages of the pre-purchase examination without fault. The only comment was that, at rest, his heart dropped a beat. This happened with absolute regularity after every seventh beat, and the phenomenon disappeared when the heart-rate increased with exercise. Quite a high percentage of horses have been found to show this 'regular irregularity', so that it is considered to be an acceptable physiological peculiarity, rather than a pathological disorder.

After purchase, Solitaire went to live at a busy livery yard. The owners requested regular health checks for the horse because they were relatively inexperienced. However, on monitoring the heart-rate it was found that far from it being slow with a regular dropped beat (as it had been on purchase), in the new environment it had a consistent resting rate of 45 beats per minute, the very top of the normal range. What brought about this dramatic change was almost certainly the level of noise, which was considerably greater in the new home.

Solitaire had exchanged a non-reverberating, peaceful stable for one made of hollow, clanking tubular steel, with sliding doors on metal runners, swivel mangers, drop catches and a blaring radio. The increase in heart-rate suggested that he was now living in a state of perpetual anxiety. It began to affect his movements. His back became more and more rigid, which increased the concussion to the front feet. It was not long before degenerative processes in the forefeet were suspected, and the owners began to consider a claim for permanent loss of use.

It might seem preposterous to suggest that the tension caused by environmental noise could culminate in such significant wear and tear on a horse's limbs. However, some years ago, an experiment was demonstrated on television, which showed how sensitive the horse can be to outside

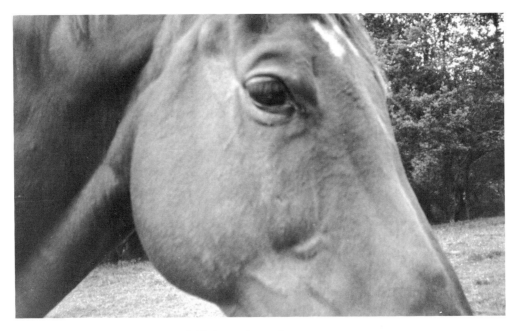

Without the ears, the intention of this horse is unclear.

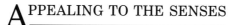

(a)   (b)   (c)

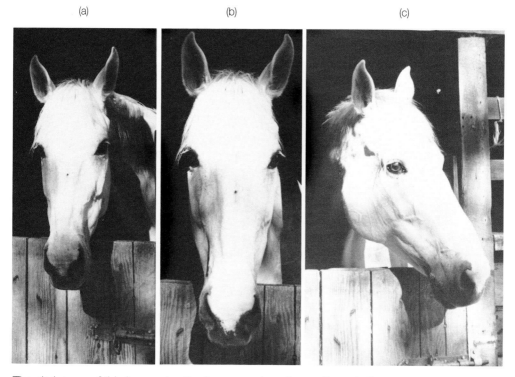

The dark eyes of this horse give the face an enigmatic quality; only the ears and the direction of the head indicate: (a) mild interest; (b) alert attention; (c) slight scepticism.

influences. A young, recently broken-in horse was to be saddled and then ridden by two different riders, one experienced, one novice. The heart-rates of both riders and horse were monitored. When saddled by the confident rider, there was little change in either horse or rider. However, the novice rider was apprehensive, and when it came to his turn, both his heart-rate and that of the horse increased significantly.

Although in extreme cases, we now consider noise to be a form of pollution, we have generally come to accept that most of our everyday activities are accompanied by a constant background of sounds, most of which are man-made. Advertising, for example, would be unthinkable, without its associating jingles.

Music

It is not known when the first music was created. The earliest example of a musical instrument, a clay ocarina, dates from about 10,000BC. Music is a very ancient form of communication and, all over the world, mythologies give its creation as either divine or supernatural. It is part of rituals and ceremonies in every culture. The ancient Egyptians said that music had

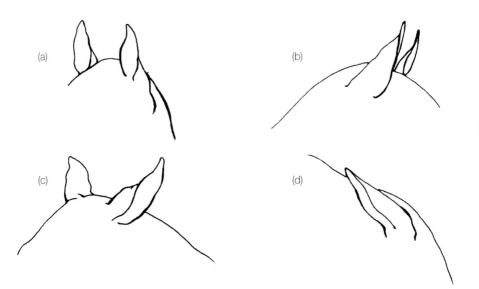

The position of the ears changes the outline of the head, and the signal can be seen from a distance: (a) alert; (b) focusing; (c) peaceful); (d) not to be messed with.

a two-fold influence over man: a physical sensation and an emotional one, like a spell. The Chinese believed that music had the power to sustain universal harmony, and that there was magic power in sounds.

Music was used for healing. Thousands of years ago this was probably in the form of a wordless wailing and specialist healers emerged, who used monotonal and rhythmic singing in their rituals. This is the basis of Shamanism, which survives in the native tribes of the Americas and in parts of Africa, Australia and the South Pacific islands.

Equestrianism has its own long-standing musical tradition. The horse was once a military animal, and music traditionally accompanied the soldier into battle. With its particular choice of outdoor instruments, the military march, for example, could affect a whole military unit at once, heightening concentration, unifying movements and focusing the emotions. The harmonies and rhythms of military music are bright, brisk and brassy. Their sentiment is still expressed in the notes of the hunting horn, to which horses, and humans, respond with animation.

How much the horse responds to melody is difficult to evaluate, but he is certainly susceptible to changes of rhythm. For this reason, music is an

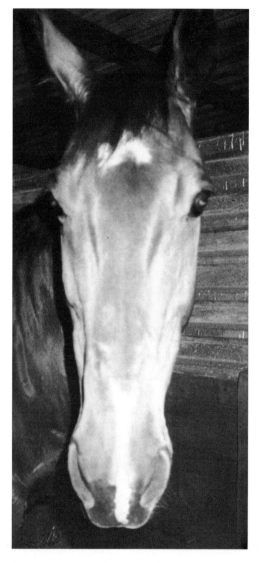

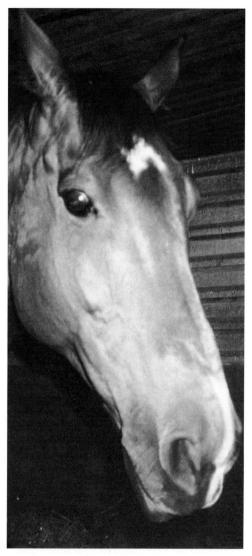

The eyes appear to concentrate, but it is the ears that are paying attention.

Eyes, ears, and nostrils together express slight apprehension.

excellent means of correcting or improving gait imperfections. In work carried out with horses and ponies belonging to an R.D.A. (Riding for the Disabled) group, it was found that, when moving freely on the lunge, they would naturally adjust the gait to the rhythm of the music, changing from trot to canter and back as the beat demanded, rather than obeying the verbal commands. Vivaldi's *Four Seasons*, with its concise and rhythmically characteristic episodes, lends itself very well to these sorts of transitions. Dressage to music has achieved respect and admiration at top competition level, with some performances memorable enough to rival those of ice-dancing. At lower competition level, the horse's sense of rhythm is

Levels of Hearing

There are different levels of hearing. It is possible to block out certain sounds, preventing them from reaching the conscious level; or else to filter specific sounds that we want to hear out of a general hubbub. This takes place on the other side of the auditory nerve, in the brain itself. However, we can only close our psychological ears, not our physical ones. Horses can appear to turn a 'deaf ear', but they probably never really shut down their sense of hearing. A horse lying flat out in a field can appear almost dead, until you look at his ears, which will twitch in response to the sounds of his environment. Furthermore, the horse registers frequencies that are beyond our hearing range. There is no way to regulate incoming sound. If we want to give our eyes a rest, we close our eyelids. If, as humans, we want to close our ears we can put our hands over them, but very often we close them indirectly, by tensing the jaw, the scalp and the neck muscles.

sometimes surprisingly handicapped by his test music, when the otherwise familiar beat is fractionally changed by being played on different equipment. The well-rehearsed balance previously mastered becomes a shuffle or a scuttle to keep in time with the music.

Radios are often heard in stable yards, and there is no reason to suppose that horses are the least bit judgmental about the sort of music they hear. Nevertheless, different radio stations use different frequencies, depending on the intention of their transmission. Serious discussions are emphasized by lower frequencies, while popular music uses higher frequencies to keep us moving physically. Most stable chores are not done to Wagnerian operas or Brahms' symphonies.

It is worth considering that the horse's range of hearing may make him uncomfortable with the sort of frequencies which *we* only think of as an aid to mucking out. Conversely there may actually be health benefits in listening to other types of sound. As part of a therapy project, horses with behavioural problems were introduced at a home for children with emotional and behavioural problems. The children had to take responsibility for the care of these rescue cases. When the horses were first re-introduced to ridden work, it was found that for highly nervous horses, the slow movement of Mozart's Clarinet Quintet could turn a frenzied canter into a level-headed trot.

The human voice is also an auditory force to be reckoned with. Many horsemen instinctively talk to their horses, to calm them down or give them encouragement. Some horse owners overwhelm their equines with complex verbal reasoning, which is certainly not particularly productive, but horses *are* very quick to learn single, well-defined commands. The voice can be a powerful instrument. We have only to think of the specially selected vocal sounds that are chanted in mantras and that are capable of altering brain-wave patterns. Voices can also have an edge to them, which can make horses nervous or fidgety. When one such horse was shod, his owner was always sent away to make cups of tea because the horse would otherwise just not stand still.

Sound cannot travel in a vacuum, but neither is it restricted to travelling only through air. Every substance can be made to vibrate in sympathy with a sound source. This includes all the substances of the body, especially water. The body is made up of a lot of water, not only as part of the bloodstream and lymph fluid, but

SOUND SUMMARY

1. Sound is a form of energy. It is transmitted in the form of sound waves, which vibrate at different frequencies.

2. All substances, including biological molecules, are thought to have a natural resonating frequency.

3. The sensory organ for sound is the ear. The outer earlobe of the horse has a characteristic shape. It is moved by twenty-two, albeit very tiny, individual muscles. This allows the horse to move his ears in a 'ball-and-socket' manner, and enables him to locate sounds with great precision.

4. It is known that dogs and cats hear sounds of higher frequencies than do humans. It is assumed that horses do, too. Loudness is another feature of sound that needs consideration. Measured in decibels, zero is the threshold of hearing for humans, whilst 120 is the threshold of pain.

5. It is not possible for the ear to stop receiving sounds, even though the information may not reach the auditory cortex and be consciously heard. Sound may cause tension in the voluntary skeletal muscles or else stimulate the involuntary nervous system unnecessarily, with increased activity in inner organs.

6. Stable acoustics affect horses. Fixtures and fittings may produce uncomfortable resonances, as may traffic, machinery, radios or even voices.

7. Sound can be used therapeutically. Both the human voice and music can have a calming or animating influence on the horse.

8. Riding to music, which has a sympathetic but supporting rhythm, is a valuable training aid. Skilled choice of music can make the repetition of movements smoother, which encourages suppleness in muscles and joints, both in the horse and rider.

9. Inner organs may have individual resonating frequencies. These change with illness.

10. A change of frequency is also a change of energy. There are forms of alternative therapy that make use of certain types of sound to restore this energy.

inside and around every cell. Different tissues of animal bodies have been used in the making of musical instruments – bones, sinews, gut – all chosen for their elastic and resonant properties. In other words, sound does not enter only through our ears; we hear sounds with our whole body. This is how it is possible for musicians to be deaf.

The horse was not designed to be a cave dweller, and it may well be that his experience of sound is more intense, in the confines of his stable, than it is out in the open field. If we imagine the posture of the alert, attentive horse, the curve of his topline ends at the very tip of the ears. The hearing is primed, the muscle tone is increased, pulse and breathing follow. When the moment of interest passes, he relaxes, puts his head down and goes back to grazing. The ears move loosely, the muscles are mellow. Thus, we can understand how sound can affect a horse's sense of well-being, and how the sounds of his environment can have a 'healing' effect, just as they can – as in the case of Solitaire – a detrimental one. Sound is an energy of the universe, and music is the arrangement of sound, but we cannot appreciate either of them unless we can spare a little time for the sound of silence.

TASTE AND SMELL

Diet

It is said that the Roman emperor Caligula fed his favourite horse a diet that contained raisins, almonds and honey, and gave him diluted wine to drink out of a golden bowl. Today's horse might be partial to beer, chocolate bars, or even fish-paste sandwiches, but his working diet includes soya, peas and beans, and his water, usually chlorinated, is drunk out of a galvanized trough or a plastic bucket. Does this mean that the horse can be specially motivated by appealing to his discerning palate, or is he really just an adaptable dustbin? Is he an epicure or simply an omnivore?

Archaeological evidence shows that the forerunner of the horse, the tiny *Eohippus*, browsed on foliage. As his descendants moved on to the grassy plains, their teeth and gut had to undergo modifications in order to make use of the available foodstuffs and compete with ruminants. With domestication, the horse became horsepower! His engine needed the equivalent in fuel to the requirements of his work. This energy had to be concentrated into the daily rations of the working horse. It had to come from readily available sources, yet it did not have to overload the comparatively small equine stomach, nor upset the microbial digestive processes in the hind gut. These criteria have been the basis of equine feeding practice ever since.

Cereals were introduced to horses as long ago as the 14th century BC when exact rations of wheat and barley were apportioned to war horses according to the level of their training. Thousands of years later, in the early 19th century, the Prussian army was experimenting with cooked cereals in the form of rusks; and during the First World War pressed feed-blocks weighing up to 22lb (10kg), containing hay, oats, brewer's grains, soya, peanuts, sesame and molasses, constituted the German cavalry's 'iron reserve'. It seems that whatever man puts on the menu, the horse can be persuaded to eat.

It is something of a contradiction that on the one hand the horse is naturally highly selective in his grazing habits, while on the other it shows a complete lack of discrimination in having no apparent instinct for avoiding harmful substances. He will crave ragwort, the consumption of which results in irreversible liver damage; and I know of one pony that ate his way through a bag of cement – and survived. Probably many more horses take unpalatable medication in their feed than do refuse it.

Taste and Smell Receptors

A large part of our 'insides' really belongs to the world outside. Both the respiratory tract and the digestive system make up a large part of our insides. In the horse the surface area of the lungs is about the size of a football pitch, and the gut would just about fit into a bath tub. Lungs consist of many small tubes that end in tiny air sacs, and the digestive system is one continuous tube with several 'U' bends and an opening at either end. The surface lining of both comes into immediate contact with the outside world, via the air we breathe and the food we eat. The walls of the respiratory and the digestive system are an interface. Not only this, but they keep one another informed on the status of all incoming substances, whether inhaled or ingested.

One of the reasons for soaking hay is to make mould spores swell, so that they stick to the hay fibre and are swallowed rather than breathed into the lungs. Yet some horses still cough. The defensive tissue in the gut has passed the information about the presence of these allergens to the lungs. In fact, everything that enters the gut for the first time is regarded as a poison. It is only on the second encounter that the immune cells in the gut decide whether or not a substance is acceptable. This is why there are some foods that simply don't agree with us, even though we would really like to eat them.

Nature, of course, doesn't allow potentially harmful substances to get right to the core without a challenge. The senses of taste and smell are early-warning systems; their sensory input constitutes the first line of defence.

Perceptions of taste and smell in humans are very subjective, and they are mainly discussed in relation to food and drink. Taste is classified into four broad categories: sweet, salty, acidic and bitter. There are no such strict definitions for the qualities of smell, and their description often relies on quite poetic elaboration. The points of reference for human taste and smell are not necessarily applicable to horses. In experiments on humans it is possible to stimulate the taste and smell receptors with specific substances, measure the degree of receptor activity, and infer how these substances are perceived by a recipient. Very little work of this kind has been done with the horse.

The receptors in the nose and tongue are specific cells, which are activated by chemicals. These trigger off a change in the cells' electrical activity. The electrical impulses are passed along nerve fibres to the brain: smells to the olfactory lobe and taste to the thalamus. The thalamus is a central sorting office for all incoming messages to the central nervous system. Recognition of specific substances probably depends on the frequency of the signal, and this depends on the concentration of molecules at the receptor site. In the case of smell the molecules have to pass through the mucous layer in the nasal passages to make contact with the sensitive hair extensions of the receptor cells. In the case of taste the substances are not effectively recognized until they have been diluted in a liquid or saliva. In both cases, changes in the concentration of molecules can alter the perception between pleasant and unpleasant, or even lead to two totally different interpretations of the same substance.

The Purpose of Taste and Smell

Cuisines around the world have understood how to manipulate the human senses of taste and smell by the use of aromatic herbs and spices. In many cases these not only heighten the sense of expectation of the food, but are also an aid to the physiology of digestion. Stimulation of the olfactory nerves and the taste buds increases the activity of secretory glands all along the digestive tract.

However, taste and smell are not there only for the benefit of the digestive system. There are other physiological processes which depend for information on the activity of these senses. It is often described how animals can 'smell' danger.

This implies that the body is in some way forewarned, and can prepare itself fully for flight. Foals demonstrate this behaviour when they are investigating their new surroundings. They sniff and then nibble at unfamiliar objects, only to leap away in an instant before the object 'sniffs' back. The typical postures of sexual communication between mares and stallions are initiated by the smell of pheromones. Indeed much of the daily communication between horses is based on the combination of posture and smell.

As well as the nerve endings which are especially adapted for taste and smell perception, the nose and tongue also contain nerve fibres from other sources. These pass information associated with taste and smell to the nerve centres of the locomotor system. There are twelve major nerve systems in the head area which are made up of several different types of nerve fibre: sensory, motor and involuntary components. The optic nerve, the auditory nerve and the olfactory nerve all belong to this group of twelve. Most of the sensory information around the head area is collected by the trigeminal nerve. This has chemically sensitive fibres in the mucous membranes of the nose, and one of its subsidiary branches is linked to the taste buds in the mouth. Information is passed by this nerve to an area of major importance in the brain called the *Formatio reticularis*. Like a central, computerized, railway signal-box, this co-ordinates and integrates all the reflexes in the head, so that, for example, we don't try to swallow and breathe at the same time. It also regulates the breathing rate and blood circulation in the body, as well as forming links with the cerebellum, where movement patterns are stored, and the spinal cord, along which movement patterns are transmitted.

Using Taste and Smell in Healing

There is a form of alternative therapy called Applied Kinesiology. It is based on the idea that there is a link between taste and smell recognition and the performance of a certain muscle in the body. Substances are placed on the tongue and the resistance of a certain muscle is manually tested. The strength or weakness of muscles can be modified by balancing key elements in the diet. It is also thought that the activity of hormone-producing glands like the thyroid or adrenal glands, can cause painful sites in specific muscles, and

TASTE AND SMELL SUMMARY

1. Taste and smell are often discussed jointly because of their close anatomical arrangement and the similar way that they process information.
2. The taste and smell receptors are sensitive to chemical compounds, which are translated into electrical impulses.
3. The concentration of molecules on the receptors changes the impression of smell, but completely different molecules like, for example, sugar and saccharin, can taste exactly the same.
4. Molecules that are mirror images of one another can taste either sweet or sour. Human individuals can respond differently to the same nutritional compounds when these are manufactured by different companies.
5. Relatively little is known about the equine sense of taste and smell. Palatability studies have been mainly restricted to the use of apples, carrots and mints.
6. It is likely that in the horse, the sense of smell takes precedence over taste, though his perception of food may be mainly influenced by texture.

7. There is additional sensory information from the areas of taste and smell through fibres of the trigeminal nerve. This nerve has connections with an important area of co-ordination in the brain, which is responsible for breathing and circulation, and has further links to the locomotor system via the spinal cord.
8. Applied Kinesiology is a method of diagnosing dietary imbalance by testing skeletal-muscle response. It may have a useful role to play in diagnosing metabolic problems relating to the utilization of vitamins or trace elements in the horse, especially where dietary levels appear to be normal.
9. Stabled horses need good ventilation without draughts. Pockets of stale or stagnant air may not only be unhygienic, they may actually alter the function of internal organs and the locomotor system.
10. A ride through a pine forest, a gallop along the sea shore, the turn-out on spring grass, all these are tonics for the horse and rider.

that this activity corresponds to the influence of certain dietary substances. Gland dysfunction and its dietary adjustment is assessed according to the skeletal muscle response. In humans, caffeine, nicotine and refined sugar are examples of test substances.

Experiments are carried out to investigate the effects of inhalation on the musculo-skeletal system, using specially prepared vapours of homoeopathic remedies, Bach flower remedies and even heavy metals. Aromatherapy combines massage with the use of plant extracts and essential oils, linking the activity of internal organs to the stimulation of smell and the manipulation of muscles.

The effect of dietary substances, their aroma and their chemical contents on the athletic performance of the horse are largely a matter of speculation. Most horse owners know whether or not their horses tolerate oats or barley. Some horses respond temperamentally to the sudden release of energy from substances which are digested in the stomach, and it is now possible to avoid this problem by feeding rations that contain complex starches or oil and have a slower release of energy.

However, given the sheer diversity of ingredients which now find their way into these rations, along with the extensive use of herbs, synthetic vitamins and flavour enhancers, our categorization of feed as heating or non-heating would seem to be inadequate and simplistic. Energy concentrates for horses are not cheap, but we still have a lot to learn about the real cost of their ingredients.

TOUCH

The most direct way to influence the horse is through touch. The contact between man and horse is based on touch. Every part of the horse's education depends on his acceptance of the human hand: the foal that lets us put on the foal-slip, picking up and picking out the feet, grooming, bitting, smoothing the way for the saddle or rugs, tending wounds; every aspect of the horse's care involves the skilled and sympathetic use of touch. The partnership between horse and rider unites the horse's sense of touch with our own.

We take it very much for granted that the horse should accept our physical contact without objection. In fact, most of the areas of the horse's body which come into human contact are those that the horse probably considers to be most vulnerable. There is a famous painting by the 18th-century artist George Stubbs, which depicts a white horse being attacked by a lion. The horse is in a frenzied pose, his head and neck thrown back towards the lion, which is perched on the horse's back, biting into the withers and clawing into the ribs and quarters. The part of the horse's body being assaulted covers roughly the area of a blanket clip. In the wild this would be the area most difficult to defend against the attack of a powerful predator. We should therefore expect the horse's most basic instinct to make him particularly guarded about our own interference with this part of himself. Yet he learns to tolerate the throwing on of rugs, the strapping up of a saddle, and the shifting weight of a rider, to distinguish between caress and aggression, by virtue of the information that is passed to him through his skin.

The Skin

The skin is made up of different layers. What we see is only the uppermost surface through which the hairs grow and which provides a weatherproof barrier. Actually it is more like the sea of roofs found in an English city suburb, complete with rows and rows of chimneys, TV aerials and satellite dishes, beneath which are thousands upon thousands of electronic receivers, televisions, radios, videos and telephones. The skin even has its own utility services, in the form of blood vessels and lymph channels, which supply fuel and allow drainage.

The top layer of the skin is called the epidermis. It receives a continuous supply of cells, which become hard and horny as they die off and which are then sloughed. The depth of this layer varies according to the mechanical pressures that it has to withstand. The uppermost cells may be dead but the process of renewal is not. This is a valuable indicator of local general health. There are two layers below the epidermis, the dermis proper and the subcutis. The latter is very much the skin's basement, a storage area for fat, a service area for pipes and cables which deliver blood, lymph and nerve fibres. The sebaceous and sweat glands have their boilers in the basement but their exits are through openings in the epidermis.

The dermis houses the electronic processing equipment. This is made up of many different shapes of sensor, which transmit information about contact, pressure, vibration and temperature. The sensors are linked to nerve fibres, which are bundled together to form nerves, and which stretch as far as the spinal cord. Here they make connections with other fibres, forming loops of communication, back to the place of origin, or relaying collected data further on, up to the brain. The sensors are called receptors, and are sensitive to mechanical influences or changes of temperature. Hair roots are also linked to nerve fibres, which measure the way in which the hairs are moved. Hair loss that is caused by rubbing tack, for example, is certainly not just a cosmetic defect. The body will have already made a mental note of the unwelcome pressure and be preparing its own response, whether this be in increasing the horny layer of protection, or changing the muscle tone underneath.

All these receptors have a certain tolerance. This is why we can wear clothes or the horse wear a saddle in the first place. As long as the body can make a physiological adjustment, changing the blood flow, increasing sweat production, making hairs stand on end, the integrity of the skin is protected. An American anthropologist has written: 'The skin itself cannot think, but its sensitivity is so great ... that for versatility it must be ranked second only to the brain itself.'

The sense of touch is made up of *all* the information registered by *all* the different types of receptor. Whether the touch is smooth, soft, coarse, hard or ticklish, the feeling is arrived at by consensus. There is another group of receptors sensitive to chemicals. These are the pain receptors.

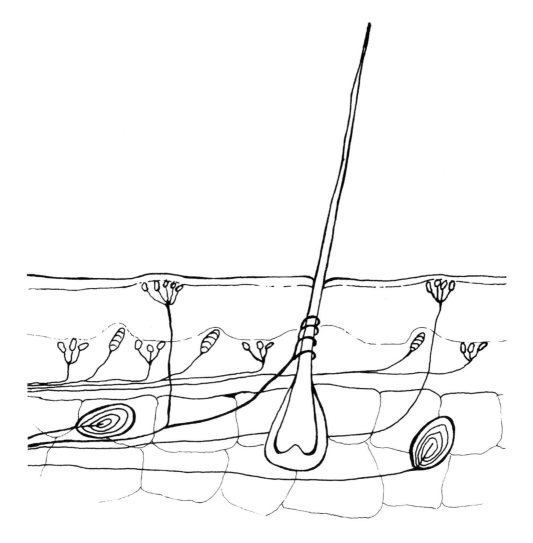

A cross-section through the layers of the skin with the relative position of a hair. The skin and the hair is 'wired' at every possible level.

Their fibres find their way to the spinal cord and form many cross links, before eventually reaching the brain. When the tolerance of any other receptor, mechanical or thermal, is exceeded, chemical sub- stances are released which warn of poten- tial damage. This triggers a response in the pain receptors. The ultimate reaction is for the whole body to move away from the harmful influence.

It is worth considering that the mechanoreceptors have a well-defined shape and size. They are rather like peas under the skin. As long as they stay whole and round, they are effective transmitters. They will stand up to a certain amount of pressure but can be badly damaged by excess wear and tear, when their usefulness is diminished considerably. There are instances where horses that have worn badly fitting saddles over long periods of time still show apparent pain when a correctly fitting saddle is used. It is possible that the mechanoreceptors have been damaged beyond repair, and that the pain receptors are being stimulated directly.

Restoring confidence in the touch of the saddle may well depend on the restoration of the pressure-sensitive structures.

The skin is a two-way communication system. It tells the inside what's happening on the outside, but it also lets the outside know how the inside is feeling. Many horses are very sensitive about being groomed. The skin may ripple with ticklishness, or it may become tense with irritation, or we might simply get booted. The skin passes the information from its surface back to the brain, which instructs the nerves and through them the muscles with an appropriate response. The co-operation between touch and muscle response is quite obvious

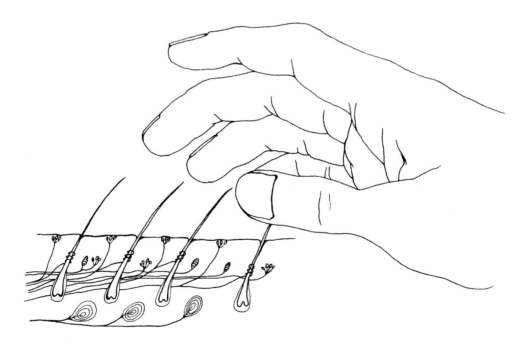

The sensors and their nerve fibres are activated by touch.

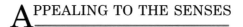

if you have ever tried to walk through a dark room without falling over the furniture.

Touch as Therapy

Touch can be used therapeutically. The sensitivity of the horse's entire body surface makes him especially receptive to all forms of therapy that are based on the sense of touch. Massage is the skill of using touch to manipulate specific areas of underlying tissue. Those professionally trained in its use learn to combine different degrees of pressure and movement of their hands for specific effects. The fingers and the patient's skin move as a unit, working the muscle or connective tissue underneath. The intention of massage may be to treat injury or to prevent it. In any event, it increases the blood flow and mobilizes the mechanical parts.

In the case of injury, the body has a fairly random way of 'gluing' together the damaged parts. This often results in undesirable adhesions between types of tissue which are really meant to glide smoothly past one another. These adhesions have to be broken down before the full range of movement can be restored. Overworked or undertrained muscles can become locked; the elasticity of the whole muscle can be compromised by the presence of small areas of spasm, which form as a result of lack of energy or fuel. The enormous muscle bulk of the horse means that sites which would potentially benefit from massage are sometimes six or ten inches (15–25cm) below the skin's surface. The pressure required to knead away lesions at this sort of depth could be damaging to the tissues above. Instead, massage uses a knock-on effect. The skin co-operates as a mediator. Its receptors interpret the forces of the massaging hand and amplify them to the brain. The lesion is then treated in two ways: by the direct stimulus of the hand and by the central response as instructed via the skin.

Everybody has used massage at some time. If a child bangs its knee, the first thing we do is rub it better. If we get sore muscles or aching joints, we use our hands to ease them. Even internal pain is reflected somewhere on the body's surface and we instinctively use our hands to relieve it. Pain is produced by the release of certain chemicals in the body's tissues which irritate specific nerve endings. Yet the body is powerfully equipped to overcome pain. It can produce its own potent pain-killers, called endorphins.

The practice of 'twitching' the horse, which involves applying a tight noose to the upper lip, is known to stimulate the release of endorphins. A horse susceptible to this method of restraint appears to go into a kind of trance, with half-closed eyes and a low drooping neck. This seems to be accompanied by a deep relaxation, which allows us to overcome the horse's apprehension. Like all methods of restraint, the twitch can be applied in a sympathetic or a heavy-handed way, and this latter has affected its reputation. Yet there is no doubt that if used correctly, the stimulus of twitching the upper lip appears to induce a response throughout the whole body of the horse.

Massage stimulates endorphin release. Since it increases the blood circulation too, it allows the drainage of waste products accumulated through injury, as well as the influx of pain-relieving and healing substances. Deep relaxation is something we humans appreciate, and animals would appear to have a similar capacity. When the dog stretches out by the fire, the cat basks on the sunny wall, or the foal lies flat out in the summer pasture, the complete absence of effort and release from tension is obvious.

Equestrianism has two 'e's: one for exhilaration and the other for exertion. In every equestrian activity we take command of the horse's movements. Even quietly hacking round the lanes makes demands on the horse's musculo-skeletal system, since the horse has to adjust his balance to include the weight of the rider. Neither horses nor humans are machines, and although we all strive for perfect harmony between horse and rider, we do have to be realistic. After the exertion and the exhilaration, we definitely need to put the 'e' back in ease.

Certain people who have worked both in training horses and in the field of sports medicine, have discovered that between the gentlest pat of the hand and the most energetically kneading fist, there are many gradations of touch which can effectively relax or stimulate the horse. Jack Meagher,

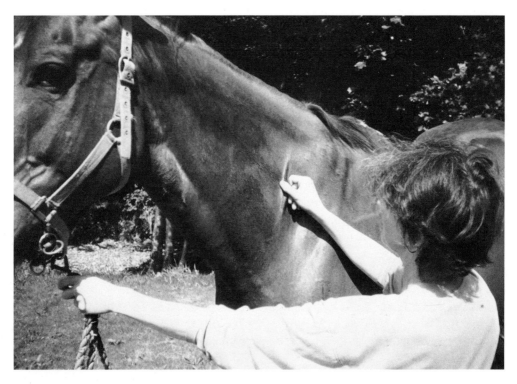

Touch can stimulate the release of endorphins by different methods. a) Pinching the skin.

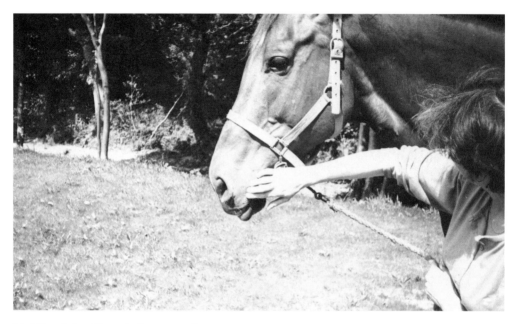

b) Stimulating fibres in the upper lip.

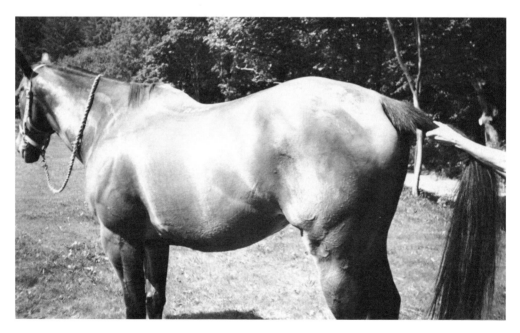

c) Gently pulling or massaging the tail.

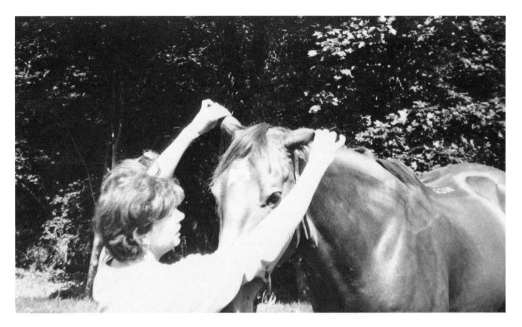

d) Stroking the ear lobes.

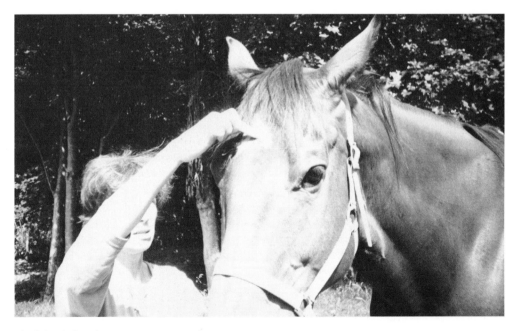

e) Stimulating the acupuncture point.

an American sports therapist and trained masseur, found that when the horse's muscles went into spasm, the site of the spasm was most commonly near the muscle's point of origin. Since these spasms appear to be concentrated into a localized area of muscle, he has called them stress points. The stress points produced vary according to the discipline in which the horse is working, but their overall pattern is remarkably consistent. They can be relieved by massage.

As might be expected, these points are often painful. The recommended pressure for massage is 5–10lb (2.3–4.5kg) of thrust, which is not always tolerated by the patient. Instead, small circular movements of the finger with a very light skin contact can be used on these stress points with remarkable effect. The horse starts to blink, makes chewing movements and the eyelids and head start to droop. The neck gets longer and he seems to fall asleep. As long as there is

TOUCH SUMMARY

1 The sensation of touch is conveyed to the brain by specific receptors in the skin. The sense of feeling is the result of contact, pressure, vibration and temperature.

2. Particular areas of the horse's body are especially sensitive to touch: the head, the coronary band, the frogs, around the sheath or vulva.

3. The information from the mechano-receptors is thought to override any stimulus of the pain receptors. If they are damaged or destroyed then the pain receptors dominate.

4. High levels of pressure produced by uneven flocking in a saddle will eventually cause a painful response when the body can no longer respond to the information of the pressure sensors.

5. Endorphins are the body's own pain-relieving substances. Their production is implicated in all forms of healing, and stimulated by many forms of alternative medicine.

6. Massage encourages endorphin release. The frictional massage required to break down some adhesions may be painful, but the stimulus can be applied below the pain threshold.

7. Massage is a skill which requires training. If it is being used for a specific therapeutic purpose, it should be carried out by a qualified physiotherapist.

8. Every horse owner can increase his contact and knowledge of his horse through the sense of touch. The feel of the skin, and the quality of the tissue beneath it, are reliable indicators of the horse's well being.

9. The simplest form of massage is grooming. It not only prepares the horse physically for work, but also tells us how the horse might be feeling emotionally; calm and relaxed, or 'a touch irritable'.

10. We can develop our own awareness of touch, by looking at the horse's response. We can learn to use it effectively, like a person playing a musical instrument. Touch is the basis of many alternative therapies. In fact, it's the very gateway to them.

gentle stimulation of one of these points, the horse is quite oblivious to irritation by flies or noise. The same effect can be achieved with tail massage, which has the additional advantage of stretching the long back muscles. Linda Tellington-Jones has developed these methods in her own form of healing, which does not confine the massage to Jack Meagher's stress points. The Tellington Touch is used to calm nervous horses in behavioural therapy, and in preparation for strenuous competition, as well as for relief after exertion.

The sense of touch has many dimensions. A horse can plaster himself all over with mud, but he can also feel the tiniest fly on his quarters. Touch is a powerful communicator; it has the potential to harm, but more importantly it has the power to heal.

Grooming

The general trend for clipping horses out in winter and then protecting them with a stylish wardrobe of rugs, is labour-saving. Nobody likes to be faced with an hour-long task of removing half the field from the coat of their horse before eventually climbing into the saddle, especially on a cold winter's night after a hard day at work. Yet, undoubtedly the horse is missing out on a thorough groom as the most valuable part of the preparation for his ridden work. Grooming is massage. It stimulates the blood circulation, loosens the back and increases the muscle tone. Picking out the feet, we gently flex the joints and mobilize the joint fluid. Asking the horse to step round with a light touch of the finger on the lower rib cage, introduces the communication of touch which is the foundation for our riding.

4
MANIPULATING THE SPINE

The breaking wave
And the muscle as it contracts
Obey the same law.

An austere line
Gathers the body's play of strength
In a bold balance.

Shall my soul meet
This curve, as a bend in the road
On her way to form?
                Dag Hammarskjöld, '*Single Form*'

Manipulation is probably the most commonly used form of alternative medicine in horses, yet its consequences are far from being properly understood. The methods are more diverse, the application more controversial, than any other form of treatment. Every horseman has, or knows where to get hold of, a 'back person'. Human medicine has come to accept back manipulation, and equestrian sport has come to depend on it. Nevertheless, the veterinary profession tends to regard it with scepticism, distrust and, in some cases, downright dismay.

Is everybody who has used, or advocated the use of manipulation for their horses, really being taken for a ride? Is it possible to re-align the horse by banging about on some prominent bones? Was the horse asymmetrical in the first place? Does it even matter?

Western medicine, as we know it, is still comparatively in its infancy. It seems to be so advanced only because science and technology have given us highly sophisticated precision instruments for both surgery and diagnosis. Yet the concept of modern medicine really began with the awareness of hygiene and the development of disinfection, and this didn't happen until the beginning of the nineteenth century. The idea began to establish itself that disease was caused by an agent. This eventually led to the discovery of antibiotics, since without having formulated some notion of the existence of germs, there would have been no necessity to look for a substance that would kill them.

Antibiotics are used in types of infection caused by bacteria, but other causal agents, like viruses and allergens, have since been discovered or at least hypothesized. The concept of a causal agent is reasonable enough for the understanding of infectious, allergic or even some cancerous disease processes: a harmful agent is identified as an intruder, while the body is considered to be a helpless victim. However, there are two areas of medicine where this formula simply doesn't work, and those are in the treatments of headache and back pain. Unless either of these problems is associated with actual organ dysfunction, for example, headaches from eye problems, migraines from blood pressure imbalance, or back pain from disc degeneration, the responsibility for the disorder cannot be passed on to an outside agent. At the moment Western medicine avoids the issue, transferring the formula of elimination on to the pain itself: hence pain-killers. Other cultures have also had to deal with the phenomenon of pain, but none has stopped the development of its medical thinking at this point. All other forms of medicine have progressed towards the philosophy, that the basis for treatment is *not* what the disease does with the body, but what the body does with disease.

Back pain is not new. It must have existed for all the ancient cultures, since they all place so much philosophical importance on the physical well-being of the spinal column. In medical traditions that are now some 2,000 years old, the spine is the focal point for life-giving and

healing energy. Every organ disorder can be detected as energy imbalances along pathways that run parallel to the backbone. Not only the physical integrity but also the spiritual development of every individual is regarded as being dependent on the free flow of energy along the back. After just 200 years, it is possible that Western medicine still has a long way to go before it will be able to recognize back pain as anything more than just an enigma.

The fact that the human animal walks in an upright position is often held to be ultimately responsible for the development of pains in the back. Contributing factors are thought to be unequal posture, caused perhaps by having one leg shorter than the other, or a one-sided muscle spasm, or discomfort from an internal organ, or else compressive forces which cause wear on the discs, the collapse of vertebrae, and the squashing of nerve roots. However, the upright-walking human also has a mental anatomy, and this influences the posture of his spine a great deal. For example, if you feel on top of the world, or it's just a bright sunny day, or you have a particularly positive approach to a problem, you will walk in a very different way from a person who is bowed down with anxiety or depression. Our everyday language is full of images that suggest we intuitively know how much our spines are put upon by the state of our emotions: we talk of something being like a millstone round our necks, or we feel a great weight has been lifted from our shoulders.

Looking at the extremes of pressure and deformation which the back can withstand if adequately trained, as it does in athletics or gymnastics, the average back should be strong enough to cope with the daily activities of the average human being. Yet the free flow of movement is significantly altered by emotional states. The calm of confidence, the thrill of expectation, or the tension of anger or anxiety all modify muscular activity. The real pressure on the human spine is pressure from within the mind.

THE SPINE

Whether you are a human or a horse, the anatomical components of the back are the same. They consist of bone, ligaments, muscles, tendons and nerves, along with the connective tissue, fat, blood, and lymph and spinal fluid. The solid central structure of the back is the spine. It is made up of bones called vertebrae, which are basically all shaped like thick, bony rings. Different sections of the vertebral column have extensions to these rings of different lengths, which provide attachments for the muscles in that area. This gives each group of vertebrae a typical appearance for a particular section of the back. In the horse the most pronounced of these extensions are the ones that reach vertically upwards, called dorsal spinous processes. These give the horse's characteristic top line with its saddle-inviting profile.

The spine has two functions. It provides a central axis for the skeleton, and it houses the spinal cord. The spine is a continuous tunnel, made up of segments of bone, each of which have a 'service exit' between them. The spinal cord itself is made of nerve fibres. These are extensions of nerve cells, which are housed in, or very close to, the brain. The extensions may travel a few inches, or several feet, in order to reach their intended exit. At each exit there are junction boxes. From here some nerve fibres relay information back to the brain about the state of the exit hole itself, while others connect up with nerve fibres going to the peripheral muscles, or to separate collecting points for the nerves which control the internal organs.

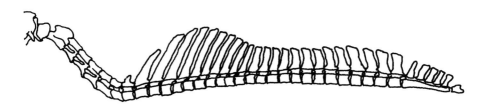

The spine of the horse showing the different directions of the dorsal spinous processes.

There are practical reasons for having several junctions in the length of one nerve. The whole body, but particularly the musculo-skeletal system, has to be able to bend and stretch. If a single continuous fibre had to reach all the way from the brain stem right down to the bottom of the horse's hind leg, for example, it would need a vast amount of extra length to accommodate all the variations in movement. By dividing the nerve into two or three shorter sections, the relative extremes of movement are allowed for by the joins.

Apart from the service exits, the segments of the spinal tunnel are strapped tightly together by ligaments, so that the spinal cord, which is after all a continuation of the brain, cannot be damaged by untoward movement. Together with small interlocking bone extensions, the ligaments keep the vertebrae in line. If, for any reason, these ligaments are overstretched or weakened, this alignment can be put at risk. The width of the service exits may be changed, resulting in compression, or fraying of the nerves. There may even be consequences for the continuity of the whole spinal cord, leading to severance of the nerves and causing paralysis.

Muscles are the working parts of the musculo-skeletal system. They are bundles of contracting fibres which are attached by passive extensions, the tendons, to two different bones which move in relation to each other. Muscles are not autonomous. They only do as they are told and it's the nerves that tell them. If there is no command, then there is no muscle contraction.

The horse's back appears to be flexible, even though a great deal of the spine is not. The neck vertebrae are obviously able to take part in a great range of movements, but the degree of flexion between any of the other vertebrae is, in most cases, less than half an inch (1cm) in any direction. When the horse rounds his back, or yields to the rider's leg, the arch or curve of the back is achieved almost solely by the outline of the muscles.

There is one hinge in the back. This is between the last vertebra of the loins and the first vertebra of the quarters. A

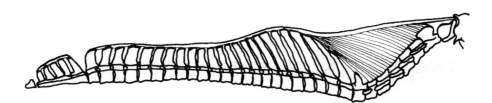

The horse's spine showing the nuchal ligament, which is called the supraspinous ligament when it attaches to the top of the dorsal spinous processes. It ends at the lumbosacral junction to allow for considerable flexion of the pelvic ring (lowering the quarters).

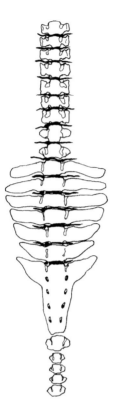

The vertebral column showing the service exits for the nerves (full length of nerves not shown).

processes would be unable to stay upright. The degree to which the horse can flex his pelvis depends on the long back muscles, which start either side of the spine at the pelvis, and continue on the left and right side of the spine to the withers, where they pass under the shoulder blades to the base of the neck. If the horse has a constitutionally broad back, or has powerful back muscles through training, this hinge mechanism will be efficient under saddle, and well protected from strain. If the long back muscles are weak or undertrained, the hinge will be very vulnerable, susceptible to injury, and extremely painful.

Anatomically speaking, the term 'back' is taken to mean the thoracolumbar spine. In the horse it consists of those vertebrae which begin at the withers, continue under the saddle and end at the beginning of the quarters. Functionally, however, the back cannot really be isolated from the rest of the body. The horse's head and neck are of great importance to the carriage of his back, and the movement of his tail will tell us a lot about his back's comfort. The supraspinous ligament which is attached to the dorsal spinous processes from the lumbar spine through to the withers, also spans from the withers forwards to the base of the skull. This part of it is called the nuchal ligament, and it can be tensioned like the single string of a primitive instrument by increasing the flexion of the neck vertebrae. The changing tension here is passed right along the ligament, eventually applying traction and support to the spine behind the saddle. The ability of the spine to lift itself, whilst being propelled forwards by the muscles

strong supporting ligament, called the supraspinous ligament, which attaches to all the dorsal spinous processes as far as the last lumbar vertebra, ends at this point. A new ligament begins with the first element of the sacrum. The hinge allows the horse to lower the pelvis sufficiently – whether for a piaffe or a pee! This avoids overstretching the supraspinous ligament, without which the dorsal spinous

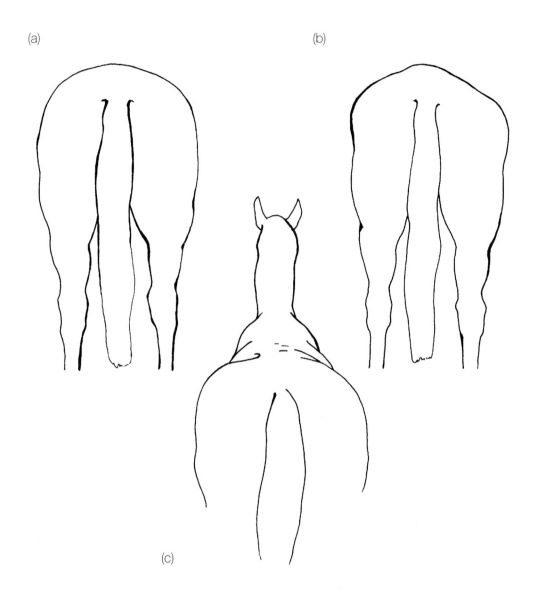

(a)

(b)

(c)

The symmetry of the horse's quarters depends on the fixation of the skeleton, and the way he uses the muscles. (a) Symmetrical; (b) skeletally out of line; (c) One-sidedness: muscles of one side that have developed more than those of the other side may hide a skeletal problem.

of the quarters and the back, depends very much on the correct 'tuning' of the nuchal ligament.

The thoracolumbar spine is positioned between the four legs – one at each corner. It is suspended between the shoulder blades at one end and by the pelvic ring at the other. Any condition or activity that affects the movement of any limb, including shoeing, affects the balance of the back. If the condition, for example, stiff-ness, lameness or foot imbalance, persists beyond more than a few days, the back will begin to behave as a counterweight, or prop. Sometimes the change in normal movement of a limb can develop so slowly that the back is continually making small adjustments. This compensation can be so habit-forming that the back itself becomes 'lame', and continues to be so, long after the original limb problem has been cured.

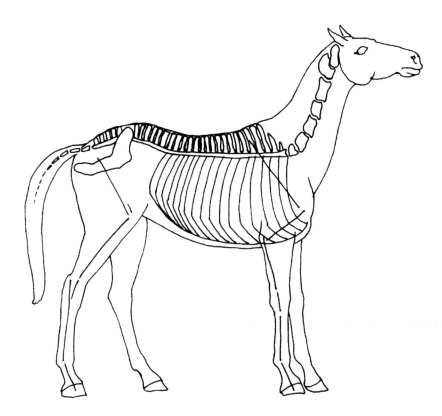

The effect of hollowing the back on the position of the dorsal spinous processes. Horses may spend long hours in this position if they have to reach for their hay.

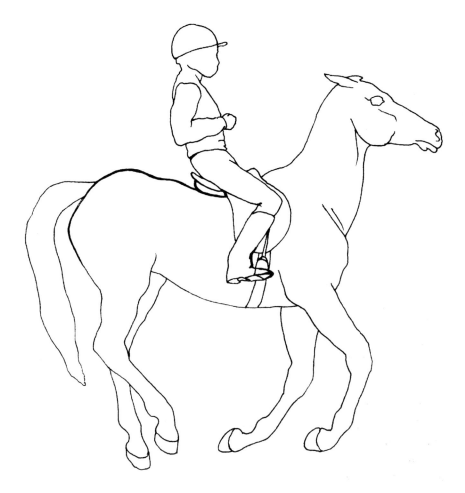

The effect of hollowing the back under the rider on the position of the dorsal spinous processes can only be imagined.

BACK DISORDERS

The disorders that affect the horse's back fall into two categories: back pain and back problem. The terms are often used synonymously, but wherever possible we should try to make a clear distinction between the two, since this helps us to be more specific in the choice of therapy.

Back Pain

Pain occurs when there is even so much as a hint of damage to any type of tissue. The types of tissue that make up the structures of the back are no exception. It may be that pain is less easily suppressed here because any damage potentially threatens the function of the spinal cord. Inflammation causes pain around the extensions of the vertebrae if these are constantly rubbed together, for example, or around ligaments that are overstretched. These ligaments may be reinforced with deposits of bone material and this process is also painful while it is active. Blood vessels, especially the small capillaries, can become squashed, depriving tissues of fuel. In the case of muscles, areas with insufficient blood supply have to rely on recycling their own energy products. An accumulation of waste materials from this source is potentially damaging to the muscle tissue. Nerves can be compressed, so that the impulses no longer reach their destination. Nerve fibres have a protective soft tissue sheath, which must remain intact for the nerve to transmit at the correct speed. This, too, is subject to inflammation when there is undue wear.

Pain is probably a way of summoning help. The damage is signalled by the release of chemicals, which irritate specific nerve endings. Messages are transmitted to mobilize the necessary work force, but not all of these messages reach the conscious brain: minor repairs are carried out all over the body without the individual being aware of them. The perception of pain, and its tolerance, vary enormously, not only in different species but among different individuals of the same species. It is often said that horses have a low pain threshold, that they can't put up with pain, or that they are wimps. However, some of the conditions that are revealed in the course of lameness investigations, can have more than a sobering effect on the riders when they consider that the horse has been ridden, and even competed, with conditions that are presumed to be extremely painful.

Back Problem

The back problem, on the other hand, may not be a fault of the back itself, and may not even be painful if there is no actual tissue damage. There are many situations in which the horse has to use his back to compensate for imbalances elsewhere. It could be the result of having to work on difficult ground, a rough hard surface, deep slippery sand, or the steep camber of a road. It may come from the imbalance of the feet, or the shoes, or the stiffness in one joint. The head and neck are extensions of the back, and are an integral part of its movement. Artificial restriction of these will impose restrictions on the fluency of the back movements.

CAUSES OF BACK PROBLEMS
The shape and fit of the saddle can cause the horse's back anything from a mild problem to severe and chronic pain. The saddle was developed thousands of years ago, and was an invention of necessity for use in battle. Light weapons could be used by a horseman riding bareback; only when weapons became heavier or needed more thrust, as in the lance or the great longbow, did the rider need a safe anchorage on the back of his horse. The saddle was invented as a means of staying on.

The basic idea of saddle construction has not changed much since that time, although the demands on the horse in modern forms of competition have changed a great deal. In all forms of equestrian sport, a high level of precision is required, which depends upon the accuracy of the commands given by the rider, largely through the saddle. It might be argued that precision riding has always been a sporting feature to accompany the military use of the horse. However, the shape of the horse in today's competition differs greatly from the shape of the horse used even 300 years ago. The lean, eventing Thoroughbred, and to some extent the flat-quartered Warmblood have a back construction that is not supported in the same way as that of a Baroque dressage horse, or a mediaeval war horse.

Saddle design is at last being rethought. It is moving away from the original concept of clamping a large, more or less upholstered, wooden 'peg' to the horse's

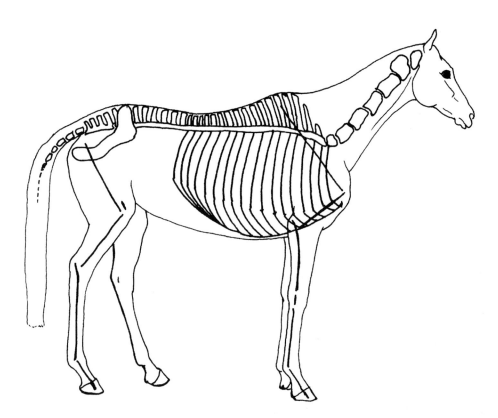

The position of the skeleton in the horse's body.

withers, and then strapping it as tightly as possible around his chest. It is now recognized that the saddle can cover a greater area of the horse's long back muscles, giving a greater area of weight distribution for the rider, while still allowing the horse to move relatively freely underneath.

The way in which the rider sits in the saddle can also be the source of a back problem. If the rider sits with 50 per cent of his weight on either side of the spine, then the horse should be able to move symmetrically. If the rider sits more to one side than the other, for example, 60 per cent on one side and 40 per cent on the other, then the weight ratio now differs by 20 per cent, which is quite considerable if you are trying to produce the same quality of movement on the left and right rein.

Riders often ask how much weight a horse can carry. There is obviously an upper weight limit for every horse, but the deciding factor is how far back the rider sits and where the weight is placed along the length of the back, in relation to the supporting and moving parts. The backbone, the fixed ribs and the breastbone form a cage, which is relatively static and can therefore support a load. Behind the saddle the vertebrae are unsupported except by ligaments, long external back muscles and two very much shorter internal ones. There is nothing between the lumbar spine and the ground apart from the gut. The rider who has long legs, but rides short, or the rider who is really too tall for the horse sits partly or wholly on the unsupported spine. The consequence is that the horse hollows away from unwelcome pressure, is unable to make use of

the traction on the supraspinous ligament to lift the spine, and therefore has to rely on the long back muscles for support, when these should be engaged in moving him forwards.

The rider's legs, correctly placed, encourage the horse to lift his abdominal muscles. The tensioning of the abdominal muscles increases the supporting strength of the spine. If the rider's legs have insufficient or no contact with the side of the horse, then the abdominal lift is exchanged for the weight of pendulous tummy.

If the pelvis is not level, the muscles either side of the spine will function unevenly, giving the rider the impression that one side of the back is lower under the saddle than the other. The pelvis is attached to the spine by two large slabs of bone which are stuck to matching extensions of the first element of the sacrum. The two parts are joined by strong connective tissue. Together they form the sacro-iliac joint. It's called a joint because it is a junction between two bones, but it is a joint which is not supposed to articulate. The sacrum and the pelvis together form a ring, within which lie vital internal organs. In the horse the stability of this ring of bone is protected by the powerful muscles of the quarters. If there is the slightest risk of dislodging the sacro-iliac joint, through a slip or a fall, the muscles immediately clamp onto the bones to stop them being shunted out of place. A very severe fall or jolt can displace the bones, with tearing of the soft tissue fibres in between. Nevertheless, in many cases, the muscles lock the bones just as they reach the limit of their normal range of movement. The

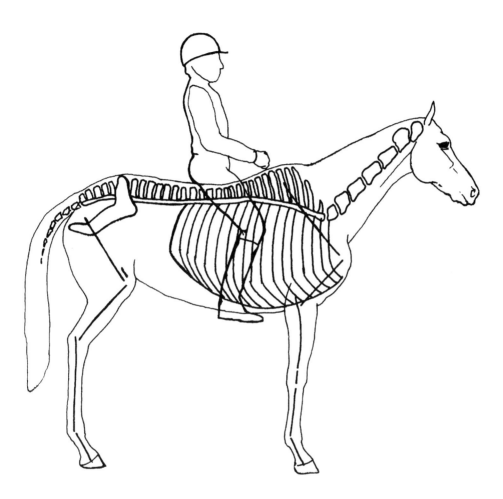

The position of the rider relative to the horse's skeleton – there is little skeletal support behind the saddle.

muscles remain contracted, holding the pelvis in this position until something, or someone, tells them to do otherwise. This condition can exist for years.

True sacro-iliac strain, as opposed to muscular spasm, is probably extremely painful when it first happens, and is certainly accompanied by severe lameness.

Eventually the join is recemented with strong fibrous tissue, and the skeleton is stabilized. The pelvis remains at an angle with various consequences for horse and rider. The horse may adapt his body movements to the tilt of the pelvis. He will be permanently fixed in that bend, regardless of the rider's aids. This can be thought of as a back *problem*. However, the horse may try to compensate for the tilted pelvis, by tilting his head and neck in the opposite direction. This causes the first neck vertebra, the atlas, to become fixed at a similar angle to the pelvis, but with an opposing slant. If a line is drawn from the most lateral point of the right pelvis to the opposite most lateral point of the left atlas, and vice versa, the crossover point will usually be just behind the saddle. This is also the junction between the supported and unsupported vertebrae. This area becomes the focal point for the compensatory twist of the whole spine. It is an area often associated with back *pain*.

There are many incidents in a horse's life which can disturb the balance of the pelvis. Slipping in mud, slipping on tarmac, landing awkwardly over a jump, a car stopping too closely behind, shunting, jolting, tipping over backwards. The degree of lameness is not always a reliable indicator of the nature of the damage. The gluteal muscle may be in spasm, the sacro-iliac joint may be weakened, or there may be a fracture. (More of these are coming to light with the increased use of diagnostic scintigraphy.) Straightening out a horse with a pelvic tilt is a major part of the work done by manipulative therapists. For muscle spasm, manipulation may be the therapy of choice;

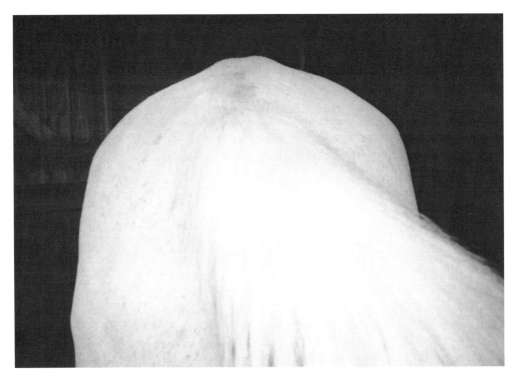

The skeletal landmarks are all out of line.

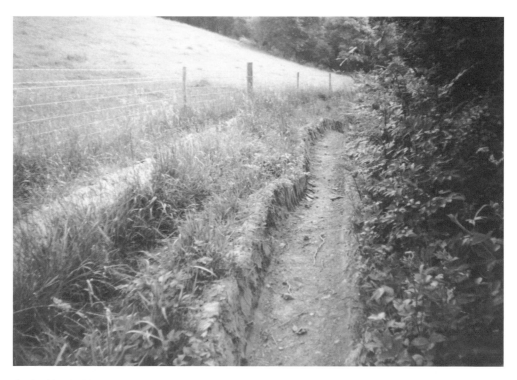

An inviting bridlepath, but a horse stepping off suddenly with a hind limb into such a deep rut might well need a visit from the chiropractor.

for chronic sacro-iliac strain, it may be less than effective; and for fractures, it is obviously downright dangerous.

Realigning the Spine

Many alternative therapies have a connection with the philosophical content of ancient medical practices. They are concerned with the imbalance in the body and the process of harmonizing the body's functions, rather than diagnosing a causal agent. In the case of manipulation, the therapist is presented with a body which

has a kink in it. In the particular case of the horse, the cause for the kink may be apparent, and a therapist with a detailed knowledge of horses may be able to advise on preventative measures. This is not the purpose of manipulation; this is simply a bonus for the horse owner. Because the therapist acts on the presenting signs, the effect of manipulation is immediate. It is this immediacy which makes this therapy so successful, so sought after, and so potentially open to misuse.

There are many different approaches to manipulation, and equally many cautionary tales about its use. Well-intentioned

(a)

(b)

(c)

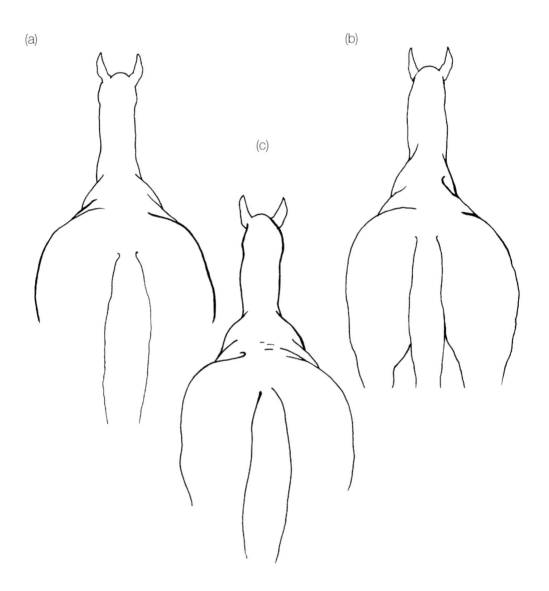

The alignment of the pelvis, shoulders and atlas bone: (a) symmetrical; (b) the right hip has dropped and there is hollowing behind the right shoulder; (c) there is tension across the loins with an uneven pull on the muscles of the quarters and compensation at the poll.

manipulators have pulled this, pinged that, pushed and shoved, heaved and hoed, even *walked up and down* on the horse's back in the name of back therapy. Bearing in mind that it is not possible to manipulate the spine without influencing the spinal cord, those that have legal responsibility for the horse's health, namely the vets, have looked on with a mixture of scepticism and horror.

Straight-laced science does concede that the horse's neck vertebrae may be affected by manipulation, and that a small degree of muscle spasm may also be released, yet there are relatively few converts among members of the veterinary profession as a whole. Nevertheless, anybody who has seen horses that previously could only move unwillingly and asymmetrically, walk away from some forms of manipulation with a 'smile' on their faces, might be inclined to judge this form of therapy as practically rewarding and very worthwhile.

The most important thing is to find out:
• what can be moved
• what should be moved
• and what is best left alone.

Without taking into account the emotional influence on movement, the musculo-skeletal system behaves like a machine. It appears to be a very complex machine, but it is, in fact, made up of very simple moving parts. It is rather like the difference between a child's nursery rhyme tune and Tchaikovsky's Violin Concerto: the one only contains a few notes, the other contains a great many notes, which have to be played very fast and often at the same time. At the end of the day, though, they are all just notes and sufficient practice will enable the player to graduate from the song to the concerto, in just the same way as a baby who is learning to crawl can one day train to be an athlete.

The principle instruments of movement are the muscles, bones and nerves. Bones are connected to each other by a variety of differently shaped, flexible joints, some allowing a straightforward to-and-fro movement like a hinge, others allowing an all-round movement like a ball and socket. Movement is produced when one bone moves in relation to another to which it is joined. Muscles have fixed attachments to bones. Since they can only contract, if one bone is static the other has to respond to the pull of the muscle. Muscles are commanded by nerves. A contraction is the response to an electrical signal. The length of the muscle is monitored by a tiny apparatus, usually within the belly of the muscles, called a muscle spindle, and its signals travel faster than those to the main muscle bulk. Information from the muscle spindle is relayed to supporting and opposing muscles so that one individual muscle rarely responds by itself, and so that, for example, the muscles do not try to flex and extend the limb at the same time.

Mechanically speaking, the musculo-skeletal system consists of passively moving parts, actively moving parts and a power supply, which for muscles and nerves comes in the form of electricity. In many respects it obeys the same laws as any non-biological machine. If the mechanical parts of a machine get jammed we can either try to move them manually, or we can try to use the power supply to do it for us. The same applies to the bio-mechanical machine: we can attempt to manipulate the bones directly, or we can try to tap into the nervous supply, and use the electrical impulse to stimulate the muscle. This in turn will move the bone. Many techniques of manipulation actually have their origins in observations from the field of engineering.

There are two main schools of manipulation: chiropractic and osteopathy. They use specialist skills for diagnosis and treatment which are based around the development of the sense of touch. The names of the two therapies describe their points of origin in the minds of the men who created them, rather than classifying two separate therapy forms. Osteopathy literally means the treatment of bones, whereas chiropractic means manipulation by the hands. Anybody who has watched practitioners of both schools at work, will know that the chiropractor adjusts bones with his hands, while the osteopath uses his hands to adjust bones! In terms of biomechanics, the starting point for osteopathy is the manual release of joints, whereas chiropractic uses the potential assistance of the electrical impulses to release muscles. However, neither school can manipulate anything without the co-operation of the soft tissues (muscles, ligaments, tendons, and their protective sheaths). Both systems of manipulation are concerned with harmonizing the whole body and both of them place special emphasis on the adjustment of the spine.

The function of the inner organs can be affected by restricted movement of the musculo-skeletal system. All internal organs occupy a space. They are covered by a slippery surface which enables them to glide smoothly against their neighbour as the body moves about. The lungs envelop the heart, the stomach glides next to the liver, the intestinal loops move up and down against each other. Each organ is suspended so that it cannot be jarred, but if one moves, they all have to: the space between is microscopic. For horses and humans, a kink, particularly along the spine, means one organ will be unnaturally compressed. This eventually has consequences for a neighbouring organ, and so on and so forth, until all the internal structures are operating under duress.

The function of the inner organs is managed by the vegetative nervous system. Although these nerves have their own command centres like the solar or brachial plexus, which lie outside the spinal cord, they still have to get to these centres along the same route as the motor nerves, that is, via the vertebral column. Therefore a kink in the back also influences the efficiency of this nervous supply to the internal organs, and thus their level of activity.

It should be remembered that *anybody* who practises spinal manipulation takes full responsibility for *all* types of spinal nerve.

The most popular word in the manipulator's jargon is 'out'. This word is really at the very heart of the veterinary profession's scepticism, because it is open to such different interpretations. Humans talk of putting their backs out: they may be referring to muscle spasm exerting a one-sided pull on a vertebra, or a slipped disc.

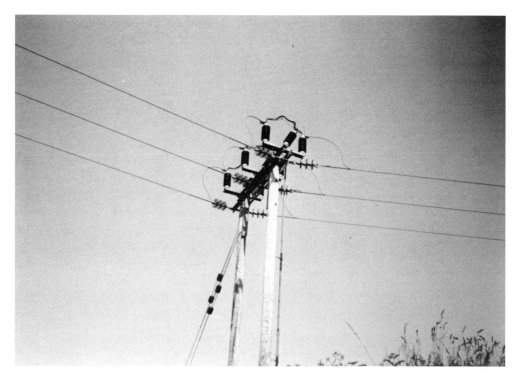

Nerves are like electricity wires: at every junction in the spine they not only relay their electrical impulses onwards, but also register information about the alignment of the vertebrae.

The 'outness' describes the misalignment of the vertebrae from front to back or from side to side. As far as we know the horse does not suffer from slipped discs, but he does suffer from misalignments caused by muscle spasm.

The manipulative therapist uses prominent parts of the skeleton as points of reference. The wings of the atlas, the dorsal spinous processes, the 'points of the hip', are among those bony landmarks which will be out of line if there is an uneven pull exerted by the muscles. The adjustment is intended to re-align these points so that both halves of the body appear symmetrical.

Veterinary medical science does not so much doubt that this is possible, but rather that it is *humanly* possible with something as large and powerful as a horse. Well, mankind built the Pyramids, and erected Stonehenge, so it is possible for humans to move mountains, even though we are not really sure how. Osteopathic manipulation of the horse's pelvis has been carried out under general anaesthetic using radiographs as a control. It was demonstrated that the alignment of bones changed. Horses with totally dissimilar left/right body halves, walk away from chiropractic with an apparently symmetrical outline.

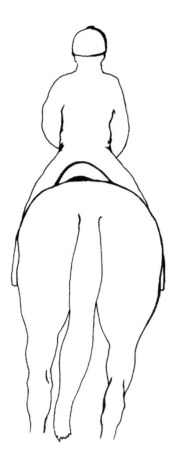

A possible candidate for manipulation: the horse is hollowing away from the left side of the saddle, causing the saddle to swing across the dorsal spinous processes. The rider sits twisted and the overall balance of the pair becomes difficult to maintain.

There are many things to commend manipulative therapy. It is quick acting and drug free. Nevertheless, it should be practised only with the following warning: manipulation means change. Usually

it is a change for the better; sometimes sadly, it is a change for the worse, but however gentle the technique, it is in the very nature of manipulation to change what it treats.

In the case of a recent injury, the change will only be one of correction. Yet it is quite possible for a joint in the limb or back to be locked by muscle spasm for years. It may begin as a very small area of restriction, after an accident or trauma, but become progressively worse as the body adapts its movements around the spasm. Even the rider may not be aware that he, too, is continually making adjustments to match the changing balance of the horse. Manipulation can still be very useful in releasing long-standing muscle restrictions. If the joints have not suffered from wear and tear as a consequence then symmetry can often still be achieved, but not necessarily balance, at least not immediately. Structures which underlie areas of restricted muscle movement – for example, smaller muscles, tendons, ligaments – will probably have been fairly inactive at the same time. Suddenly the restriction is removed and they wake up to the fact that once upon a time they had a job to do. They will obviously not be at their full strength, and need time to be retrained. Therefore, after manipulative treatment, one limb or even one whole side of the horse may appear initially to be much weaker, or even seriously lame. This situation appears on the face of it to be a change – for the worse. However, it is then possible to focus on the true cause of the imbalance, and be more specific in the process of rehabilitation. This has to be a change for the better.

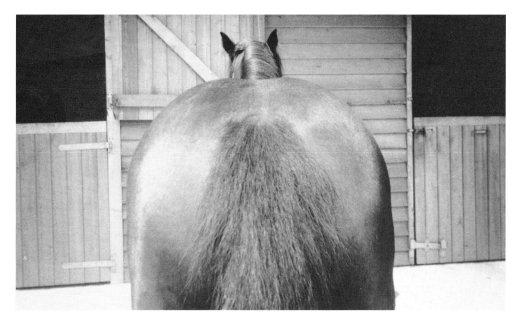

Hindquarters that are evenly muscled.

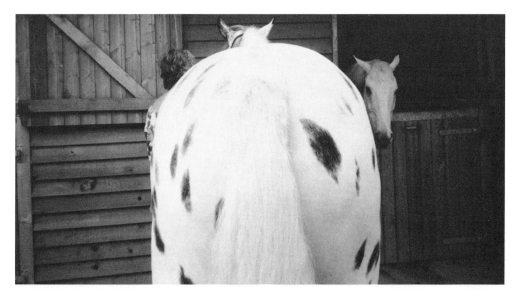

Gluteal muscles that have developed differently: the horse injured the left hind limb quite seriously some years ago. Although sound, muscularly this limb has not caught up with the other side.

The movements of the rider are strongly influenced by his emotional make-up. A happy individual would find it unnatural to slam doors or stamp up and down, whereas an angry person might move energetically but not lightly. The horse is sensitive to the presence of human emotion, even if this is not openly expressed. It affects the tension or softness of the rider's muscles and is certainly transmitted through the saddle and probably the reins. The horse's movements become a replica of the rider's. If the rider is tense, the horse will be tense; if the rider has an electrical backside, every horse ridden by that person will behave in an agitated, fizzy manner.

The horse even reproduces specific areas of restriction which the rider may have. If the rider clamps his buttocks then

SUMMARY

1. In the horse, manipulative therapy is used mainly to treat back disorders. In humans, manipulation of the spine and other parts of the musculo-skeletal system is used to treat inner health. This latter concept has yet to find its way into equine therapy.

2. The musculo-skeletal system consists of bones, their joints, and the soft tissue components, muscles, tendons, the protective sheaths called fascia, ligaments, and nerves.

3. Bones cannot be 'out' by themselves. If they are, it is because they are broken or dislocated, or their soft tissue fixation (ligament or fascia) has been damaged. Manipulation must be used here very sensitively and with precise knowledge of the diagnosis.

4. Usually if bones are 'out' it is because they are being held in that position by muscles that are permanently contracted (in spasm).

5. Releasing muscles frees other structures which have not been used for some time. These will be weak and need a period of retraining.

6. Back disorders fall into two categories in the horse: back pain and back problem.

7. Humans with back pain adopt characteristic postures, put a hand to the back or stoop. These are signals to other humans to stay away from the person in pain. A sudden pain in the back makes a person stand absolutely still. The horse may try to give signals. If he cannot stop while being ridden, he may try to bolt or nap.

8. Back problems may be caused by imbalances anywhere: the working surface, the shoes, the feet, the limbs, the teeth, the saddle or the rider. Back problems are often not painful to begin with.

9. Riding a horse with a back problem may be part of the therapy. Riding a horse with back pain is potentially very dangerous.

10. Manipulation means change. The manipulative therapist carries a great deal of responsibility, not only for the spine, but for the spinal cord and, in fact, for the whole horse.

so will the horse. If the rider does not swing through the lower back then neither will the horse. If the rider is tight across the shoulder blades, the horse will find it hard to use his shoulders freely. Every rider has areas of imperfect balance or movement. Some he will work on and improve, some may never be resolved.

The chiropractor or the osteopath treats the horse and irons out all the little wrinkles that probably weren't part of the horse in the first place. The horse, for a time, becomes his own self. It is essential that the rider understands that some of his horse's imperfections really come from himself. The success of manipulative therapy in the horse often depends on whether the rider is willing to go down the same path: to change. Many riders seem to have recognized this need, and the interest in training methods such as those of Alexander and Feldenkrais is increasing, as an adjunct to traditional riding instruction.

The techniques of chiropractic and osteopathy are less then a century old, but they are based on very ancient concepts of medicine: namely that, 'All remedies necessary to health exist in the body, in such condition that the remedies may naturally associate themselves and relieve the afflicted'. (Dr Andrew Taylor Still, founder of osteopathy.)

Whatever we believe to be the true nature of the body's healing energy, both ancient and modern therapies have associated its existence with the integrity of the spine. If the passage of this energy is to have an uninterrupted flow then the spine cannot afford to have a kink in it; not in the rider and not in the horse.

5

TRANSFORMING
THE ENERGY

'And now here is my secret,' said the little fox, 'a very simple secret: it is only with the heart that one can see rightly; what is essential is invisible to the eye.'

Antoine de Saint-Exupéry:
The Little Prince

If you place your fingers lightly on the top of the horse's spine, for example at the withers, you might feel a slight tingling sensation. It is like 'feeling' the hum of telephone wires, and it probably comes from the activity of the spinal cord, as thousands upon thousands of electrical signals pass up and down the nerve fibres. It is possible to follow this sensation all the way along the dorsal spinous processes to the horse's quarters. The tingling can vary a great deal in intensity, and can sometimes disappear altogether. Diagnosing its strength and continuity plays an important part in evaluating the health of the horse's back and even the health of the whole horse.

If you pass your hand very slowly over the horse's body, from the poll down the neck, over the rib cage, up the belly to the loins, and then down the quarters, your fingers may detect areas with markedly different surface temperatures. An area of the neck not more than a hand's breadth across may feel flat and cold, even though it is right next to an area that is comfortably warm. This finding does not depend on exercise, and is not a sign of inflammation. It is an indication of the way in which the horse's energy is distributed. This kind of diagnosis can reveal whether a horse is in touch with his whole body, or whether he has shut himself off from one part, owing to a previous physical or mental trauma.

In the course of this exploration the fingers pass over the contours of the muscles. Where muscles overlap, or in the length of one individual muscle, there will be small depressions. With practice it is possible to feel the same tingling sensation here in

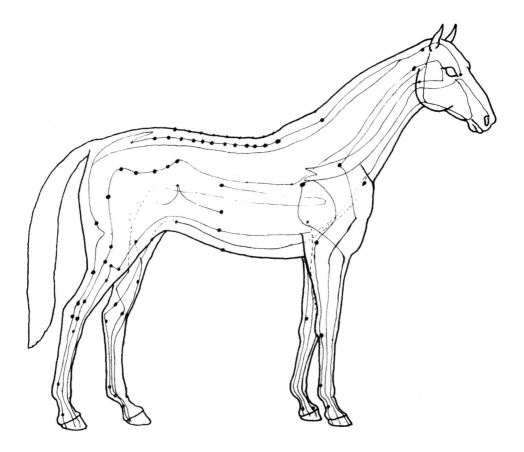

Energy channels run through the length and breadth of the horse's body and limbs. The lines here represent acupuncture channels with some of the most commonly used points for needling or laser acupuncture.

these hollows as was present along the spine. These are small areas of skin where the electrical activity of the body comes very close to the body's surface. Some of them will lie directly over nerves, others over small command centres where nerves enter muscles. They are trigger points and acupoints, and horses as well as humans have many hundreds of them.

To begin with, these phenomena simply tell us that we have, under our fingertips, a living being: a being that has certain

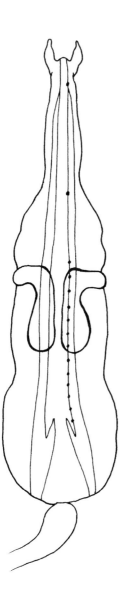

The urinary bladder channel runs parallel to the spine and therefore under the saddle. The points illustrated are used to diagnose problems emerging from other channels.

energy requirements and one that expresses that energy differently in different parts of the body. Before the invention of diagnostic instruments, palpation (diagnosing by touch) was one of the most important sources of information in medical practice. Ancient cultures of the world developed this sense of touch sufficiently to be able to influence the body's energy towards the process of healing.

Many people will find it difficult to interpret what they are feeling under the horse's skin because our conventional sense of touch has quite different points of reference. When a horse comes in lame, we instinctively feel down the leg for heat, swelling or symptoms of pain, because we have learned that these are all signs of injury. Diagnosing areas of energy imbalance in the body is very similar, except that the fingertips have to be much more finely tuned. It also helps to be able to visualize the way in which energy might flow around the body, for example in the system of energy channels used in acupuncture treatment.

Influencing the body's energy is a powerful form of medicine. It can be used alongside orthodox medicine or it can stand on its own merits. There is no reason why we should not provide immediate relief using conventional drugs, while at the same time providing the body with the energetic wherewithal for repair.

There are four basic means by which the horse owner can apply restorative energy to the horse:

1. Physiotherapy.
2. Acupuncture.
3. Homoeopathy.
4. Healing.

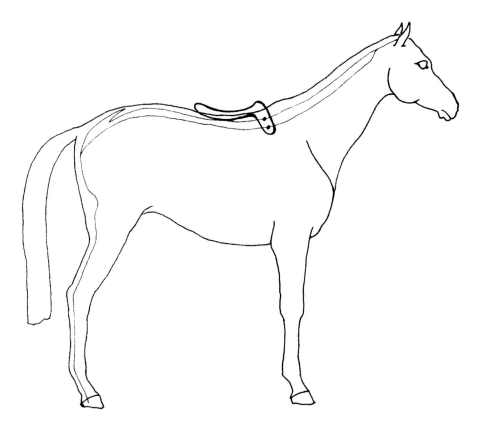

The points of the tree touch points along the bladder channel. Pain or bruising here is often associated with restricted forelimb movement and potential lameness. The acupoints would indicate the area of limb most affected by the lameness.

PHYSIOTHERAPY

There are occasions in conventional medicine where energy is used as part of a treatment: for example, malignant cancer cells, themselves a form of energy out of control, are treated with the destructive force of radiation. Yet even the most trivial illnesses can be thought of as energy out of balance, and although orthodox medicine does not do so, they can logically be treated by applying a small energetic stimulus. In ancient medical philosophies there was a common thread of belief that the cells of the

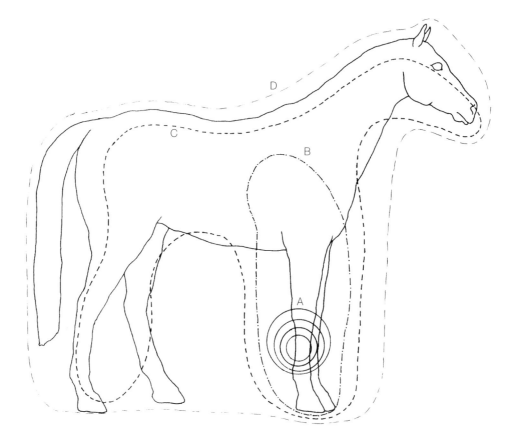

Energy medicines focus their effects in different ways. This is illustrated in a forelimb lameness: A, A physiotherapy machine concentrates its energy at the point of application; B, Acupuncture influences the energy around a specific channel; C, The energy of a homoeopathic remedy will reach any tissue in need of treatment, even if not specifically diagnosed; D, the benefits of hands-on healing suggest that the whole body is enveloped by the effect.

body were constantly vibrating, and that in illness these vibrations were no longer in harmony. The most ancient way to correct this was by using sound, originally made by the human voice. The frequency of sound imposed from an outside source raised or lowered the frequencies of the body tissues until the harmony was restored.

The concept of applying specific frequencies of energy to stimulate healing is the basis of physiotherapy. In humans physiotherapy is often prescribed as an adjunct to surgery or in addition to conventional medication, yet it is the one branch of modern medicine which has recognized that when tissue is damaged cells have abnormal activity, and that this can be corrected using different forms of energy: heat, cold, electromagnetism, laser and ultrasound, for example. In this way physiotherapy represents a link between many ancient forms of medical treatment and modern twentieth-century medicine.

In the treatment of horses, one of the simplest ways to apply energy is by cold water hosing. As the cold penetrates the tissue, it causes the blood vessels eventually to dilate, which enables healing materials to flow into the area more easily. The pressure of hosing massages the tissue, improving the drainage of waste products and helping to prevent the formation of unwelcome adhesions. Other simple means of providing an energy stimulus include stretching and flexing exercises, and small amounts of in-hand walking.

The passive manipulation of joints encourages the production of joint fluid,

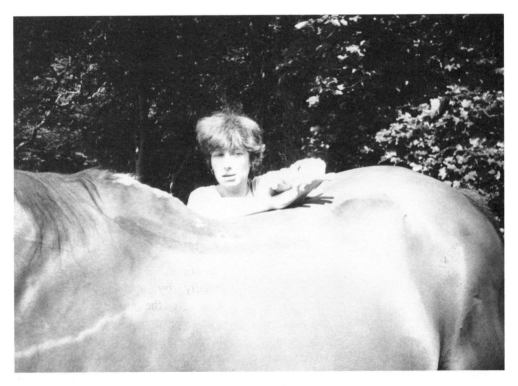

Influencing the energy balance by hand: manipulation.

while specific loading of the limbs during short bouts of exercise can stimulate the direction of repair in the cells of tendons and bones, rather than just letting them form less organized, and probably less functional, scar tissue.

The object of physiotherapy is to improve blood circulation, assist lymphatic drainage, increase mobility and restore function. In other words it tries to improve the healing process by removing blockages. This is the essence of alternative medicine. However, physiotherapy is a *modern* science and it has adapted some modern technological inventions to what are basically some very ancient forms of healing.

Physiotherapy Machines

Ultrasound is sound that is way above the frequencies registered by the human ear. It was first discovered in the eighteenth century through the observation of bats. In 1927, two scientists found that when they directed an ultrasound beam of considerable energy towards a single-cell freshwater organism, this was literally torn to pieces. The report of this experiment generated a lot of interest in the medical world, and the effect of ultrasound on biological tissue was refined until it achieved more therapeutic results. In the therapeutic ultrasound machine, vibrations are created by bombarding a crystal with a high-frequency current. The vibrations pass from the treatment head, usually through a coupling medium, into the living tissue. All the cells in the pathway of these sound waves receive what amounts to a micromassage. This has an effect on the energy of the cells, on their metabolism, and especially on the electrical properties of the cell's proteins. The use of ultrasound is, in effect, a logical extension of cold water hosing, providing the same beneficial stimulus not to a whole limb, but to a specific group of cells.

Sunlight was used to treat anaemia in humans in the fifth century BC. Yet in the late 1970s, the healing effect of laser light was hailed as magic. Nobody knew why it worked, and nobody could offer a scientific explanation for the way in which it appeared to speed up healing. Since then a great deal of research has been carried out into the effects of Low Intensity (cold) Laser Light, and it is now known that the light beam of a single wave length stimulates cell respiration. It is thought that the electro-chemical activity of damaged cells is disturbed, and that this activity can be changed by the selective energy of the laser beam. Low Intensity Laser Light is now used in wound management, treatment of chronic pain and the repair of damaged nerves.

Ultrasound and laser are not the only energy-producing instruments used in physiotherapy, though they are probably the most frequently used in the treatment of horses. Rebuilding muscle bulk was once carried out using a Faradic machine, which stimulated a muscle contraction artificially by applying an electrical impulse. If the muscle was already painful, this procedure could be painful too, and the muscle only retained its function, and therefore its size, if the nerve which served it was fully functional. It is now possible to stimulate muscle function more physiologically by applying the

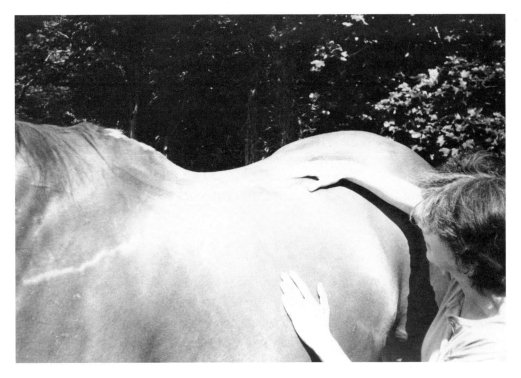

Influencing the energy balance by hand: therapeutic touch.

electrical impulse to the nerve itself, using a neurotrophic muscle stimulator.

Other types of physiotherapy machines include Magneto-Pulse, Electrovet, H-wave and Interferential therapy. Although the therapeutic energy is produced in different ways, physiotherapy machines are all variations on a theme. Energy produces heat and this increases circulation. Unfortunately the heat also limits the amount of energy that can be passed through the skin without burning the surface. While all the types of energy, Faradic-type electrical current, electromagnetism, ultrasound waves, laser light, provide a potent stimulus for healing, they

are not all suited to every type of injury in the horse.

Physiotherapy energy is man-made. Each machine uses a number of parameters to produce the energy source, and therefore this energy has to be dosed. Frequency, wavelength and intensity, as well as the characteristics of the tissue, all have to be taken into account in order to calculate the correct dose. This is best left to the professional physiotherapists!

At the moment, and very unfortunately for the professionals, physiotherapy machines can be purchased by anyone. Some unscrupulous firms actually claim that their machines can be used by people

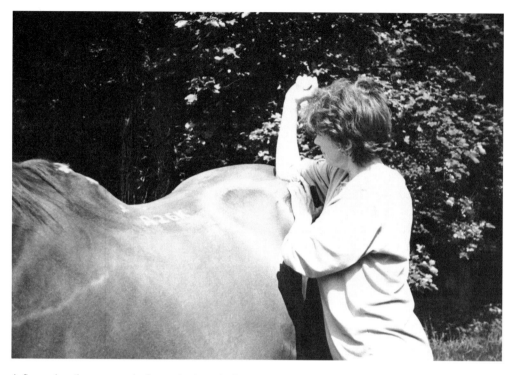

Influencing the energy balance by hand: deep massage.

with no specific training at all. Yet, however carefully we follow the instruction manual, it is doubtful whether we can ever use them as competently as a trained physiotherapist. Strictly speaking these machines should be available only on prescription, since their energy can be not only beneficial, but harmful. In particular, ultrasound machines have been used in such a heavy-handed way as to cause the disintegration of bones and severe burns to tendons.

When to Use Physiotherapy

Although specific forms of treatment should be carried out by professionals, or people acting under professional instruc-tion, it is nevertheless worth having in one's own mind a clear idea of what can or should be achieved.

As a guide, physiotherapy can be used:
1. To treat lameness after injury (especially if it persists for more than three weeks) to restore strength and re-educate the limb.
2. To treat lameness that is suspected to be of muscular origin, often difficult to diagnose and not necessarily responsive to anti-inflammatory drugs.
3. To manage arthritic pain; also to increase mobilization in older horses.
4   To treat back problems.
5. To improve athletic performance,

especially after injury or infection.

6. As preparation for and rehabilitation after surgery.

7. To restore mobilization after a long period of inactivity (for example, after the removal of a plaster cast or long-term bandaging).

8. To treat stifle problems. These joints often suffer through inadequate muscle and ligament support.

9. To break down adhesions, reduce swellings after recent injury.

10. To provide pain relief, either through stimulating endorphin release, or by working on acupuncture points via laser.

When thinking of using physiotherapy on the horse, try to answer the following questions:

1. What do you want to treat? Have you got a veterinary diagnosis or are you acting on suspicion? This may affect the outcome of the treatment.

2. How extensive is the injury? What tissues are involved? These may limit the usefulness of a particular energy type.

3. How deep is the lesion? Or is it superficial near bone or a joint surface? Again not all types of machine are suitable.

4. How much time do you have? There are often follow-up exercises which improve the overall success of the specific treatment by the machines. The more meticulously they are carried out, the better the result, but they are often time-consuming.

5. Are you planning to hire a qualified physiotherapist who specializes in animal treatment, or is it just someone who happens to have a machine? Chartered physiotherapists are insured. This is important,

both in case the horse damages the expensive equipment but also in case the equipment damages an expensive horse.

Treatment Plan

Physiotherapy treatment is a logical, step-by-step treatment:

1. Remove blockages to healing caused by stagnant damaged tissue, for example, bruising, oedema, adhesions.

2. Keep practising simple movements with the injured limb to maintain mobility. Later, increase the range of movement to as near normal as possible.

3. Strengthen the tissue by controlled weight-bearing exercises.

4. Apply energy to stimulate healing at cell level.

The above plan of treatment can be carried out in the following ways:

1. Remove blockages using heat and cold treatments, and massage.

2. Maintain mobility with flexing and stretching exercises.

3. Stimulate the repair of tissue with five-to-ten-minute walks in-hand.

4. Use a 'man-made' energy source to return cells to their normal level of activity.

ACUPUNCTURE

At about the time when people were marvelling at laser light and its effect on healing tissue, there was also renewed interest in the healing potential of acupuncture. Acupuncture had been practised for several thousand years; laser technology had only been around for a few decades, yet here again there was to be a coming together of a modern scientific invention and an ancient form of medical treatment.

Many cultures have recognized the healing properties of light, but the development of laser light enabled scientists to study the effects of specific wavelengths. During the course of this research it was found that one particular wavelength had a beneficial effect on the regeneration of nerve fibres. Treatment with acupuncture needles has a lot to do with the stimulation of certain nerve types and the production of certain chemicals, especially by the brain, in response to nerve signals. It was considered possible that this potent form of ancient medicine could be delivered by a painless beam of light. This application was especially tempting to those whose patients were horses.

Acupuncture is part of a system of medicine which originated in China. The practice of acupuncture has undergone a continuous development since it was first documented over 2,000 years ago. Strictly speaking, it should not be separated from the whole ancient Chinese philosophy of life, which is why its application in the modern western world is often a matter of very careful interpretation. For example,

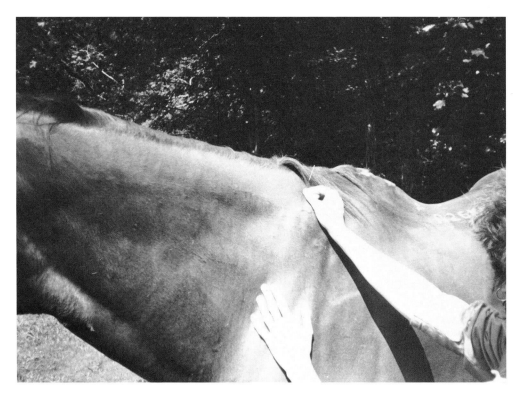

Manipulating the acupuncture needle to tonify or sedate.

the Chinese system of anatomy can be translated into Western anatomy, but the meanings of the names are often subtly different. The Chinese understanding and description of anatomy is based on function rather than on individual units. For example, we think of blood as the red fluid that flows in the blood vessels. Yet in Chinese medicine, 'blood' is not confined to precise channels but can circulate through the energy channels or meridians: it not only nourishes, but moistens all parts of the body. In Western medicine, this equates it with extracellular fluid. There are organs in Chinese medicine which have no western equivalent, such as the Triple Heater. This organ does not have an actual shape, but its function describes the relationship between the lungs, spleen and kidneys. Organs of prime importance to western medicine, like the brain and the entire nervous system are not given individual anatomical descriptions at all.

Acupuncture treatment is based on a system of channels which exists throughout the body, and which allows the body's vital energy to circulate up and down the limbs and in and out of the internal organs in a continuous flow; this circulation takes twenty-four hours to complete. Diagrams of energy channels, also called Meridians, usually show the surface channels. These appear to start and end abruptly. What they should show is that every channel enters the body at one or more points and links up with the next channel, which then returns to the body surface.

Where these channels pass close to the surface of the body, they are thought to be accessible. The channels are reached by pore-like structures in the skin, which are known as acupuncture points. The actual point on the channel really lies below the skin, sometimes a long way below, as in some of the points in the horse. If energy does not flow freely along the channels, symptoms of illness are produced. The energy is then manipulated by placing needles at certain points along its path.

This system evolved through intuition and observation, and it was eventually challenged by the new leaders after the Chinese Revolution in 1949. However, thousands of experiments and clinical trials were carried out to prove its worth and in 1958 the Central Committee decided that modern and traditional medicine should be given equal respect in China.

Western science has since carried out its own research into the pharmacological effects of acupuncture. It is known that the body can be made to produce certain chemical substances by applying needles. Endorphines, cortisol and serotonin are manufactured in certain areas of the brain and spinal cord, and their effect on the body is to relieve pain and inflammation, and alter the blood circulation. In experimental human acupuncture, these chemicals can be precisely targeted by the way in which the needles are manipulated.

The increased production of such potent substances is certainly a necessary step in the body's own initiation of repair processes. Yet the one thing research has not been able to explain is why these processes go on working long after the needle stimulation has ceased, for weeks, for months, or even for ever.

When to Use Acupuncture

There are many conditions in horses which respond to treatment by acupuncture. They are often disorders that can be only temporarily relieved by conventional medicine, or those for which suitable chemical medication is not yet available. Long-term pain relief and chronic allergies (of the skin, respiratory system, and in some forms of headshaking) pose problems resulting from long-term medication and the development of side-effects. Metabolic disturbances in the liver and the digestive system can be accurately diagnosed by modern Western methods, but there is no real Western therapy. Acupuncture diagnosis does not look at blood chemistry, it looks for certain points on the body surface which are tender. These are thought to sound the alarm for a particular organ, and the energy to that organ is then corrected by needling. This form of treatment does not give information about enzyme levels and proteins, but it is based on the observation that by needling several points, the chemistry of the liver, for example, or the digestive system, improves to the extent that the symptoms disappear anyway.

In some countries acupuncture is being widely used in horses, because it offers a therapy that is relatively inexpensive compared to long-term medication, does not involve the use of prohibited substances for competition animals, and is free from side-effects. However, the treatment itself is both an art and a science. Books on acupuncture in animals often contain diagrams of the same energy channels all with slight variations. It is a feature of Chinese medicine that no opinion is ever discarded. Therefore the diagrams are a product of the experiences of different practitioners through the ages, and they are all allowed to stand on their own merits. This is extremely confusing to the horse owner who may find that the opinions of Western acupuncturists on the location of points or the method of needling are also rather varied.

Acupuncture Methods

The horse owner who is considering having his horse treated by acupuncture should know that this form of medicine can be applied at different therapeutic levels. Again, this makes for difficulties in understanding since we are accustomed to to the idea that a pain-killer is a pain-killer, and an antibiotic is an antibiotic. They either work or they don't.

Placing a needle at *any* point on the body will generate a certain amount of pain relief. The most basic form of acupuncture is to find the place of superficial pain and stick a needle in as close to this site as possible. It is very effective, but not necessarily very durable. When the needles are placed at some distance apart along a known energy channel, a larger area of body is influenced. The effect of needling can be enhanced by twirling the needle or moving it up and down in the tissue. Treatments take place at weekly intervals, but the overall therapy is cumulative and, when it is really successful, the result will be long-lasting. Very advanced acupuncture is able to direct energy from one channel to another by using interrelated points. This is especially relevant to the treatment of the internal organs, where the energy is being manipulated via the external channel before it enters the body.

There are several methods of using acupuncture in the horse. The first is simply with the fingers. For example there is a sedating point in the centre of the horse's forehead which can be stimulated by using a small amount of finger pressure. This is a most useful way to calm nervous animals. There are points on the ears which have a similar effect. Most acupuncture points are small depressions in the skin and the trained fingertip can work the energy through these hollows. This is the basis of acupressure. Traditional needling uses steel needles which have a solid shaft with a fine point, unlike the hypodermic needles which are hollow and have a cutting edge. If the skin sensitivity is quickly overcome when the needle is applied, or the skin desensitized by a small amount of finger pressure, the passage of the needle is otherwise painless. A small amount of bruising can occur if the horse moves while the needles are in place, but this disappears within twenty-four hours. (This should be taken into account when planning an exercise routine immediately after treatment.) As the needles are placed, a horse will often begin to make chewing movements, the eyelids will begin to droop, and the head carriage will be lower. Horses often appear to be in a trance-like state, and are generally oblivious to disturbances like insects or noise.

There are several variations on the traditional form of needling. Needles can be manipulated by applying a small electric current. This has been researched in humans, since the modern approach to acupuncture is to standardize the treatment in the form of a 'dose', rather than relying on the intuition of the acupuncturist's fingers. This does not yet apply to animal treatment, which is still largely intuitive. Some practitioners warm the needles by a process called moxibustion. For this technique a wad of the herb Mugwort is ignited and held, gently smouldering, close to the shaft of the needle while it is in place. The herb gives off a pungent smell and this is thought to contribute to the overall therapy. Some acupuncturists do use hypodermic needles. Substances like vitamin B_{12} are injected at the acupuncture points where they remain as a small deposit, presumably exerting pressure on the points in the same way as acupressure. The substances are gradually absorbed into the surrounding tissue.

Acupuncture points can also be stimulated by laser light. The Low Intensity Laser has provided a most useful means of treating horses. Its depth of penetration is limited, which makes it less effective for those points that are several inches below the skin's surface, as in the horse's quarters. Nevertheless, for points on the lower limbs, which are often too sensitive for needles, laser light is more than helpful. Laser light is itself therapeutic, and it is sometimes hard to differentiate between treatment by laser, and treatment by acupuncture *using* laser. When used close to the nerves of the horse's back, for example, it is difficult to say precisely whether the nerve tissue is being healed, or whether the back energy is being healed.

Few Western veterinary acupuncturists will have actually participated in the rigorous five-year training course that acupuncturists are required to complete in order to qualify in China, so that, almost certainly, most acupuncture practised in the Western world – particularly on animals – will be a distillation of traditional principles. Nevertheless there are many conditions in the horse where the use of acupuncture, even in the simplest form, should be considered:

1. Muscle pain, bruising, soreness, or loss of muscle tone.
2. Impaired nerve function.
3. Chronic pain in, for example, developing ring-bone, side-bone, navicular disease, spavin, laminitis.
4. Inflammation in, for example, osteoarthritic conditions, and especially in the older horse.
5. Allergies of the skin or respiratory system, and also in some forms of headshaking.
6. Liver dysfunction.
7. Digestive dysfunction, poor appetite, unthriftiness.
8. Nervousness.
9. Depressed immune function, post viral infection syndrome, post strangles infection.
10. Reproductive problems.

Chinese medicine does not consist of only acupuncture. The Chinese physician would traditionally use a considerable selection of herbs to treat the internal course of the energy channels. The horseman may well be attracted to many herbal mixtures on sale through local tack shops and feed merchants. These are really only unrefined chemical substances, and very few of them will be potent energy-releasing combinations capable of complementing the effect of acupuncture. There is, however, a form of energy medicine which makes an excellent companion to acupuncture, and that is homoeopathy.

HOMOEOPATHY

' …The human body, in its living state, is a unity, a complete and rounded whole. No part can suffer without involving all the rest in suffering … and in alteration.' This was written by the founder of homoeopathy, Dr Samuel Hahnemann, a German physician in the eighteenth century who had become very disillusioned with the medical practices of his day. He began investigating other forms of treatment by translating medical texts from other cultures, and in doing so he came across the concept of curing 'like with like'. This was originally described by Hippocrates and, in fact, the ancient Romans knew that it was possible to counteract the effects of large doses of poison by taking small quantities of the same poison beforehand. Hahnemann began experimenting with this idea by applying it to known diseases. He attempted to cure them by taking small amounts of a poison which would actually cause similar symptoms to those of a specific disease. At first his experiments were disappointing, but he was not deterred. By a process of extraordinary lateral thinking, he decided *not* that the doses were too small but, were really *not small enough*, and set about finding the smallest possible dose which would cure a given set of symptoms.

Dr Hahnemann was, by all accounts, a pedantic and overbearing personality, and his family and acquaintances all became part of his system of trials to prove the effects of minute amounts of different poisons. The rigorous way in which this experimentation was carried out resulted in a catalogue of substances which produced typical combinations of symptoms, each of which resembled the symptoms of a known disease. However the work did not stop there. It was also found that by diluting the original solution of substances, tens, thousands, or tens of thousands of times, and by shaking and tapping the mixture between each dilution, the medicine increased its healing potential. This was odd because, in such highly diluted states, little or nothing of the original substance was traceable. The only explanation was that the treatment of the substance, diluting, shaking, tapping, transferred some form of energy from the solution, and that this became more and more charged, the more it was subjected to these procedures.

Today, homoeopathic preparation methods are still hotly disputed by conventional scientists, even though the concept of imprinting information, in this case on a solution, is not so far removed from other forms of imprinting which are used in computer technology or genetic science. All manner of explanations are put forward to explain the success of homoeopathic treatment, including autosuggestion. This might even be partially acceptable if it

were not for the fact that animals also respond to homoeopathic remedies.

There will always be situations where the sceptics can make a claim for 'spontaneous remission' of symptoms. Some symptoms do just disappear as quickly as they developed, and certainly horses and humans often get better without intervention from the vet or the doctor. It is good to be critical of any healing method, conventional or alternative, but there are responses to homoeopathic remedies which are entirely convincing for their own sake, which is why homoeopathic medicine is still practised.

Since there are several hundred homoeopathic remedies available, the most essential guide is a simple *Materia Medica*, a book that catalogues remedies and their most pronounced symptoms. All the symptoms are the result of 'provings', that is what different humans have experienced when taking these remedies. They are not always appropriate to horses and may have been reported by one person only. It is therefore always best to go for the most obvious symptoms first. For example, both *Rhus tox* and *Bryonia* are used to treat movement disorders; but with *Rhus tox* the movements become easier on exercise, with *Bryonia* they become worse. One old ex-riding school horse was becoming stiff and worsening with exercise. He also had a temperament that suggested the use of *Bryonia*, namely rather morose, ill-humoured and inclined to needless anxiety. He responded so well to this remedy that the mental symptoms disappeared as well as the stiffness.

Case Histories

• A twenty-one-year-old R.D.A. pony, so arthritic that his lower limbs could be flexed only manually, and already on two sachets of Bute daily, became mobile again and able to walk and trot on any surface after treatment with *Rhus Toxicodendron*. Nothing else in the management was changed.

• A foal with bastard strangles at the base of the neck, whose dam had been put down with a similar abscess entirely engulfing the windpipe, was apparently cured with Silica.

• An aged hunter, lame for three days with a large overreach wound on the bulb of the heel of a hind leg, responded to Hepar sulf. The wound, which was discharging pus, dried up and the horse was back in work three days after treatment began. The foot was not bandaged, and the horse was turned out as usual.

Homoeopathic remedies can be made from any substances, animal, vegetable or mineral. Some of the remedies are poisons, some would be poisonous if we took them in sufficient quantities. *Rhus toxicodendron* is Poison Ivy, Silica is flint, and Hepar sulf is calcium sulphide. Arsenic, strychnine, opium and cannabis all form the basis for different homoeopathic remedies. Although treatment by homoeopathy really requires a different way of looking at the presenting symptoms, it has been found that many remedies work particularly well on certain types of tissue. It is, then, possible to use homoeopathy in a way that is closer to our orthodox way of prescribing medicines. For example:

• Arnica works on the circulatory system. Both shock and bruising are different manifestations of a breakdown in the blood circulation, one generalized, one local. Both respond to this remedy.

• Symphytum is made from comfrey, otherwise called knit-bone. This remedy is an aid to healing fractures and together with Arnica can be used generally in the treatment of injuries.

• *Ruta graveolens* and *Rhus toxicodendron* make a wonderful team of remedies for treating disorders in muscles, ligaments and tendons. *Ruta* has an affinity with the tissue attachments towards the bone, *Rhus tox* with the muscles and tendons.

• *Hypericum* (St John's Wort) has a specific action on nerve fibres. Any disorder that has resulted in the compression of the nerves and their damage – in back problems, for example – can be greatly relieved by using this remedy.

Potency

In all homoeopathic remedies that are purchased, the potency will be indicated by a number after the name of the remedy. To treat acute conditions, those that have very recently happened, it is usual to apply lower potencies, often. The energy in these is not so high, but then the energy requirement of the injured tissue is not so high either. It has not been depleted by months of coping with prolonged illness. Chronic conditions need high potencies and sometimes over long periods. Some homoeopaths believe that animals generally need higher potencies than humans because their metabolism is higher. It may sometimes be more convenient to give a high potency once a day rather than a low potency every two to three hours: there are no absolute rules. The figure 6 or 30 after the name of the remedy can be regarded as a low potency, 200 or (1)M as high potency.

Strictly speaking there is no such thing as a *dose* in homoeopathy. After all, the treatment consists of an, albeit undefined, form of energy. In practical terms the remedies can be given either as tablets, drops or powders. Drops can be put in a syringe and given into the side of the mouth as for worming. Tablets or powders can be concealed in a carrot, although some substances will be taken from the hand by some horses. The most important thing to remember is that the homoeopathic remedies are vulnerable and their effect can be weakened by strong-smelling substances, like garlic and peppermint, or other herbs currently in use in horse feeds and supplements.

How many tablets is always a matter for debate, with many strict homoeopaths stating that it doesn't matter whether you are treating a hamster or an elephant, two tablets are sufficient for both. Again, in practical terms, we want to ensure that the remedy has really been received so that eight-to-ten tablets for a 15–16hh horse allows for the odd tablet being lost in the straw. (Alternatively ten to twelve drops in the side of the mouth followed by a carrot is another method.)

Homoeopathy is a means of redressing internal imbalance in the body's energy and this makes it an excellent complement to treatment by acupuncture. There are often cases which respond only half-heartedly to one or the other, but which seem to resolve completely when the two systems are used together. This applies especially to musculo-skeletal disorders and to different forms of allergy. The energized solutions of homoeopathy may act as catalysts in the healing process, or they may have specific resonances which correspond to areas of resonance in the body. This is speculation. Nevertheless their presence in the body has a knock-on effect, like dropping a pebble in a pond. Dr Hahnemann's intention was to create a form of medicine which would make waves throughout the whole body, giving any altered part an energetic nudge back to health. He applied his system to humans, but it is just as potent when used on horses.

HEALING

Closely related to the concept of homoeopathy, but originating in this century, are the Bach Flower Remedies. Dr Edward Bach was a Harley Street consultant and a bacteriologist who eventually gave up his practice to develop his own system of Flower Healing. Dr Bach's treatment was based on the idea that negative states of mind such as fear, uncertainty, over-sensitivity to ideas, or despair, drain an individual's vitality and lower his resistance to disease. He believed that anger, or depression, or any other

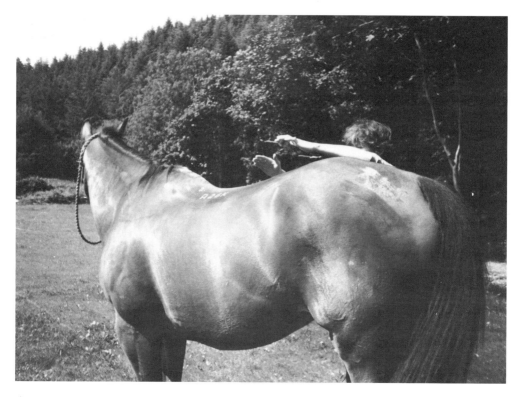

Applying healing energy.

inharmonious states of mind not only hindered recovery from illness but were really responsible for illness happening in the first place. The association between physical symptoms and strong mental characteristics had already been established in the practice of homoeopathy, where certain substances were used to treat a patient's constitution rather than the exact symptoms of disease. Tearfulness, arrogance or fastidiousness are important characteristics that are taken into account when using homoeopathic remedies Pulsatilla, Platina, and Arsenicum respectively, and may decide the appropriateness of these reme-

dies as opposed to ones that treat similar physical symptoms but do not carry such well-defined mental associations.

Dr Bach's remedies apply only to the mental states of the patient, regardless of whether that patient has been in an accident or is suffering from an illness. In his own words he says: 'Take no notice of the disease; think only of the outlook on life of the one in distress.'

It is possible to apply this concept to the treatment of horses. There are certainly horses that get angry, or that are by nature apprehensive, that have a fear of one particular thing, that are impatient, or inflexible. The difficulty lies in recognizing what is truly the horse's mental state and what mental states are attributed to it by the human partner. It would therefore probably be irresponsible to use only this form of therapy without treating the more explicit physical symptoms at the same time.

Dr Edward Bach sincerely believed in the power of the mind to heal the body's diseases and yet, quite perversely, critics of alternative medicine have attributed claims of therapeutic success to precisely this potent influence. However, without belittling any of the alternative therapies for their contribution to healing, it should never be forgotten that the *intention to heal* is a powerful force in its own right.

It is probable that every individual can exercise this power, willing themselves or others to get better. Some people refine this ability with special training, becoming hands-on or spiritual healers. They use their intuition and their hands to focus healing energy on the body of the patient. Of course, modern science does not believe in this at all, even though it is modern science which teaches us that we are all part of a complete system of energy, both terrestrial and cosmic, and influenced by these forces every second of the day.

Rescue Remedy

This is one creation of Dr Bach's which definitely belongs in every stable yard. Rescue Remedy contains five of the thirty-eight Flower Remedies:
Star of Bethlehem for shock
Rock Rose for terror and panic
Impatiens for mental stress and tension
Cherry plum for desperation
Clematis for the bemused, faraway, out-of-body feeling which might precede loss of consciousness.
This compilation is for use in emergencies, and the mental symptoms are as applicable to the horse as they are to humans.

We have become used to the destructive power of energy, which changes body tissue for the worse; why not at least theorize on the presence of constructive energy which has the power to heal.

Claims to the success of healing are usually dismissed as anecdotal, so let Dr Bach have the last word: 'Final and complete healing will come from within, from the Soul itself, which by His beneficence radiates harmony throughout the personality when allowed to do so,' and then let the horse decide.

6

THE HOLISTIC APPROACH

Look with your understanding, find out what you already know, and you'll see the way to fly.

Richard Bach: *Jonathan Livingstone Seagull*

It's eight o'clock on a Monday morning, one of the horses has torn his rug again, the children are misbehaving, you are late for work, and you've got a headache. Now you would have to be pretty single-minded, in this sort of situation, to consult the tomes of homoeopathy to decide whether the pain is worse in the morning or the evening, whether you have a prefer-ence for sea air, whether you particularly like sweet foods, whether it's a hammer-ing, pulsating or tearing pain, whether it's in the forehead or the temples, more on the left side than the right. You would be much more likely to take headache tablet. You arrive at work, the headache is forgotten, the breakfast stress is forgotten, and the rest of the day is uneventful. However, on the way home, you are driving in heavy traffic and there is a bit of a twinge in the lower back. You remember that you had really meant to call the osteopath. In the evening, picking out the horse's feet, you notice that one hind shoe is being worn unevenly, and you make a mental note to have a word with the farrier.

The greatest difficulty in establishing an holistic approach to treatment, is compart-mentalization. There is a tendency in all of us to store our knowledge in individual compartments, to have mental drawers full of facts with labels, but no system of accessing them that automatically includes cross-references. Holistic medicine is treatment which includes the individual and his mental and social situation. Even to begin to do this adequately, we have to look for a common denominator. Treating all the different bits of the horse, for exam-ple, is not the same as treating the whole horse. It is often the case that the symptoms will be linked by a common thread. The holistic approach tries to pick up this thread at one end, and unravel it, until it is eventually free from knots and tangles.

In the opening scenario, the horse wears the right hind shoe unevenly at the toe because he is stiff in the right hock. This makes it difficult for him to get up when he has been lying on this side in the stable, which is why he regularly catches the strap on his rug and tears it. He has become stiff because the weight on his back through the saddle is more pronounced on the right side. He hollows away from the pressure and therefore cannot round his back, which would allow him to step under correctly with the hind leg. The rider sits more to the right side of the saddle, because she is uncomfortable in the left hip. This comes from her place of work where she has to use an awkward posture to reach a particular machine, and unconsciously tries to relieve her back by sitting cross-legged. This, however, creates more tension across the lower back, and the twist culminates in the neck muscles, where the tension causes a headache.

In this hypothetical situation, there is one root cause for all the symptoms, namely the postural discomfort at the place of work. It is obviously very difficult to diagnose this when you are in the thick of it. Yet, what of the farrier? Has he looked at the way the horse moves to produce abnormal wear on the shoes? Has he noticed an unusual one-sidedness in the muscle development of the hind limbs? Does the horse make a fuss when he shoes one particular foot? Has the riding instructor seen the imbalance in stride, shorter on one rein, a little stiffer on one side, per-

haps? Has he discussed it with his pupil? Does the saddle seem always to be slipping to one side? Has the horse started to show signs of discomfort when the girth is done up; does he make faces? Has the saddler tried to flock the saddle more on one side than the other to balance it? Has he commented that the saddle is flocked symmetrically, therefore the problem must be in the horse? What of the osteopath? Has he asked about posture at work, or about any leisure activities?

Both in human and in equine health care, very little cross-referencing occurs. Where horses are concerned, the farrier looks after the feet, the equine dentist looks after the teeth, the backman does the back, the saddler flocks the saddle, the instructor teaches you to ride, and the vet gives injections. This gets the whole horse treated, but the treatment is not holistic. Nothing hangs together, there is no overview, no consensus.

It is in the nature of alternative medicine to be holistic. Firstly, the therapies cannot avoid treating the whole being. They work through the movement of energy, and although the therapy may be applied to one part of the body, the energy will continue to spread as far as its strength will take it. Secondly, all alternative therapies believe in the fundamental ability of the body to heal itself. They have to address the whole system, in order to find the source of the body's own healing potential. However, there are certain problems to be overcome when trying to take an holistic approach to the treatment of horses, even when the intention is to use alternative medicine.

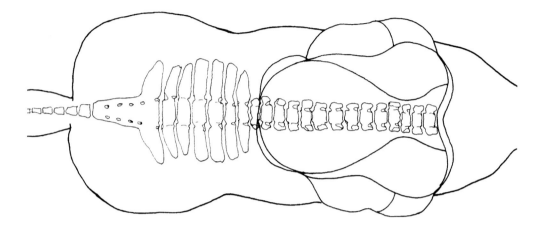

The position of the spine beneath the saddle.

For example, to treat successfully a riding horse with a musculo-skeletal disorder, it is absolutely necessary to take the rider into account. The ridden horse is locked between the saddle, with the rider in it, and the shoes, which are attached to his feet. Treating the horse holistically involves the input of the farrier, the trainer, the saddler, perhaps the physiotherapist and/or back person, and the vet – not as individuals but as members of a team. What of the horse's environment? Does he stand awkwardly because of a cantankerous neighbour, the position of his hay, or a draught? Does he get tense because his friend gets turned out before he does, because he can't see his friends at all? Is there an atmosphere of turmoil in the yard because all the horses get fed at different times? Is the owner/rider content with the livery yard? Do they come to ride after a stressful day at work? All these factors and more influence the way a horse will perform under saddle. An holistic approach to treating horses really does mean paying attention not only to the physical problem, but to the mental and social factors as well.

Fortunately, more and more in recent years, there is a healthy trend towards the teamwork among those professionals who are entrusted with the care of our horses.

Conformation and Saddle Fitting

The horse's individual conformation will significantly affect the way in which the saddle rests on the horse's back. The photographs here illustrate three of the conformations that pose particular problems for the saddler.

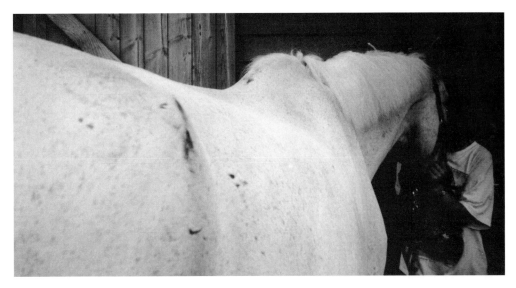

High withers and hollows behind the shoulders pose a problem for the saddler in fitting older Thoroughbred horses.

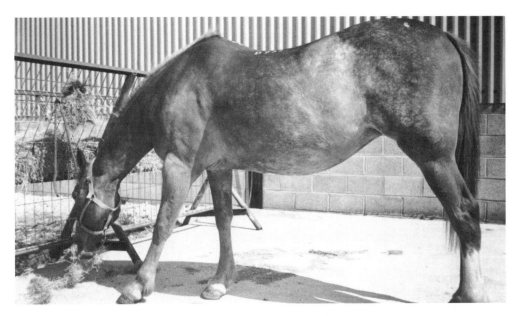

A horse with a long back and high quarters. The dorsal spinous processes are always in danger of being compressed if this horse does not lift his back under the saddle.

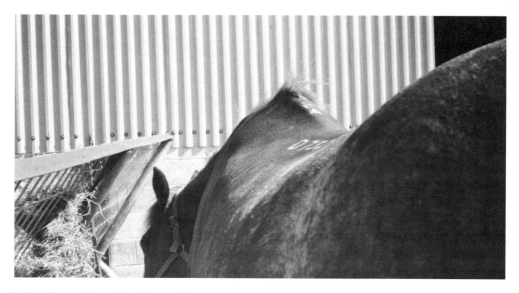

With this conformation the saddle will be prone to slide forwards, banging into the shoulder blades.

The team usually consists of a vet, a farrier, a saddler and a physiotherapist or chiropractor/osteopath. The team should include the riding instructor and the livery yard manager or groom if appropriate. Everybody looks at the horse from the point of view of his own specialization, but all the steps in the course of treatment are carried out with constant reference to how they might affect the input of the other practitioners. It can be a stimulating exchange of ideas, a creative and dynamic form of medicine, tailored to the individual horse and his special, individual circumstances. The following two case histories illustrate how the skills of different professions can be co-ordinated into a programme of rehabilitation using both orthodox and alternative medicine in combination.

A 16hh hunter-type mare was jointly owned by two ladies, who had considerable family and working commitments. They had bought the horse while they were still novice riders, but they both took their riding seriously and had weekly instruction. The mare was about twelve

Incorrect Saddle Fit

At first glance, and even on initial assessment, a saddle might appear to fit extremely well. But do not be tempted to accept that a saddler's fit is good until you have observed the way in which it is affected by the horse's assuming different postures. In the photographs here, a saddle that appears initially to be a good fit proves to be otherwise on further investigation.

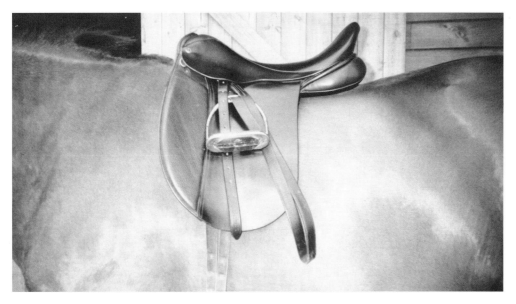

Fitting a saddle: when merely placed, unfastened, on the horse's back, this saddle seems to be a possibility.

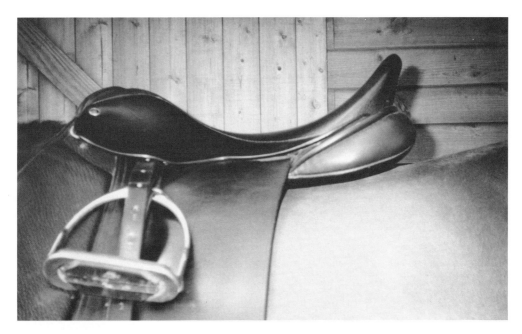

It has a generous gusset.

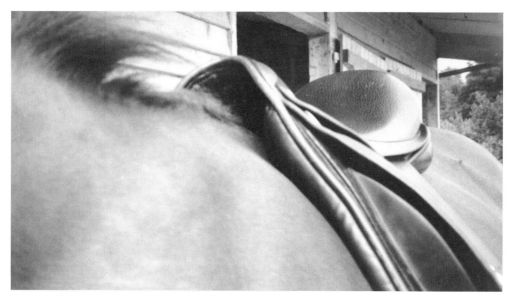

There is good clearance of the withers and shoulders.

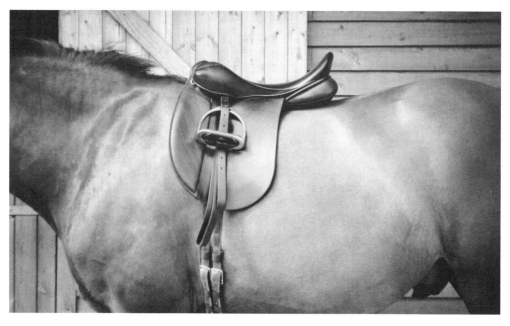

When girthed up, it still follows the contours of the back.

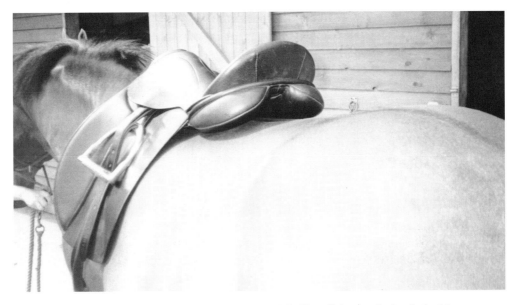

However, when the horse lowers its head, the saddle lifts off the back. It will do this whenever the rider is on board.

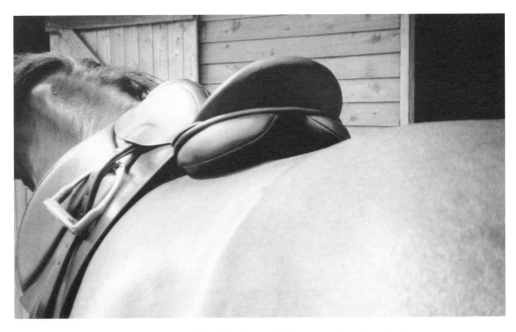

There is also movement sideways, bringing the saddle across the dorsal spinous processes.

years old and was competing in dressage and jumping at riding club level. A veterinary check was requested because the mare had a blemish on the inside of one pastern, which was a scar resulting from catching the pastern with the other hind hoof. The owners intended to show the horse that season and wondered about the implication of the scar tissue.

When the mare was led out of the stable it was apparent that she moved quite stiffly, taking short, choppy strides. The restricted reach of the forelimbs in no way matched the quite generous slope of the shoulder and the well-set-on neck. The action of the hind limbs, when watched from behind made it almost inevitable that the horse would strike a hind pastern. The leg with the scar was probably doing most of the work. The other limbs were unable either to flex or to extend correctly, depending on the gait. The back was held tightly and any palpation of the spinal reflexes was decidedly unwelcome, and obviously painful. The horse was seen lunged and then ridden. In spite of the horse's willingness, it was clearly impossible for her to keep her balance without resorting to some means of compensation. The overall picture seemed so complex and chaotic that it was decided to send the mare to a referral clinic for specialist investigation.

It was likely that each limb and probably the back, too, would throw up some sort of clinical diagnosis. By having the investigation carried out at one centre, any part of the body that was painful on palpation or flexion test could be immediately examined for its relevance by using local anaesthetic techniques and X-rays. Scintigraphy was requested, which is a means of scanning bones and soft tissue using a radioactive marker substance. With this information, the individual evidence from nerve blocks, intra-articular blocks, X-rays and muscle testing, could be put into the context of the whole horse. The mare came home from the clinic with a diagnostic shopping list. There was chronic inflammation of a ligament over one carpal joint (knee), inflammation between the dorsal spinous processes of T16 to T18 (part of the spine towards the back of the saddle), and osteoarthritis in both hocks. Navicular disease was not ruled out but the evidence was inconclusive.

Four years previously the mare had run into a car, banging the right knee. She had not seemed lame at the time, and after a brief rest to allow for any slight bruising, she went back into work. At about the same time the owners had purchased a new saddle, which fitted the horse in the shape it was then, which was rather on the narrow side, especially around the withers. The damage to the knee, insignificant at the time of the accident, began to cause wear and tear around the knee joint. The mare began to fill out around the withers, and the saddle tree became too tight. The shoulders were unable to to move freely and so the stride shortened, increasing the soreness of the knee. The narrowness of the saddle wouldn't allow the back muscles to move freely either, so that the power from the hindquarters simply shunted the lumbar spine into an area of resistance under the saddle. Since the horse could not round her back, the hind limbs were unable to absorb the concussion caused by their own movement, and the stiffness eventually led to wear and tear on the hock joints. The degree of spavin was worse in one hock than in the other, which was probably explained by its being diagonally opposite the painful forelimb.

The uneven balance between the two diagonals has its crossover point just under the rider's seat, increasing the strain on the ligaments around the dorsal spinous processes. The process of deterioration, as a result of what seemed a trivial incident, had been going on for four years. The owners mainly had riding lessons on their own horse, so that they had nothing with which to compare any loss of rhythm or difficulty in balance. They had adapted their riding to the continually changing ability of the horse without realizing it.

The clinic recommended anti-inflammatory medication and box rest for three months. The owners were doubtful about this, since they knew that the horse stiffened up even if kept in the stable for just a day. However, the recommendations were strictly followed for one week, until it became clear that the horse was so uncomfortable that confinement was unacceptable. It was decided to try to deal with the accumulation of problems in chronological order. The inflammation of the carpal joint was treated by a physiotherapist by (very cautiously) using ultrasound. At the same time, since the mare had rather boxy feet for her not ungenerous frame, a remedial farrier was consulted. The bearing surface of the front feet was increased using broad-webbed shoes, and lateral

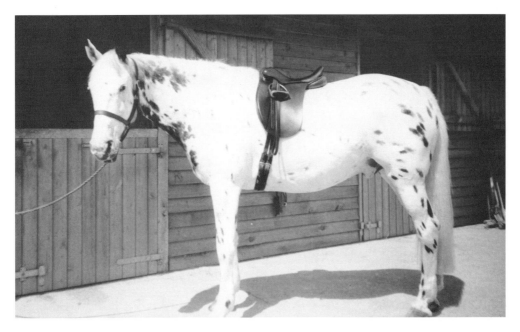

A saddle which virtually moulds itself to the muscles of the back.

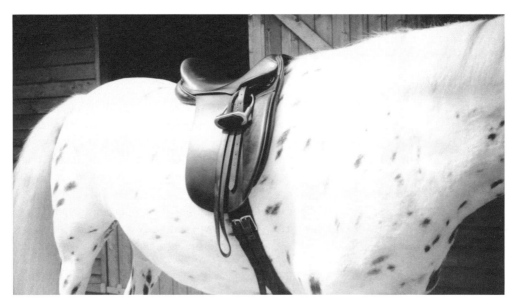

Although close fitting, clearance of the withers is maintained and the points of the tree allow freedom for the heavily built shoulders.

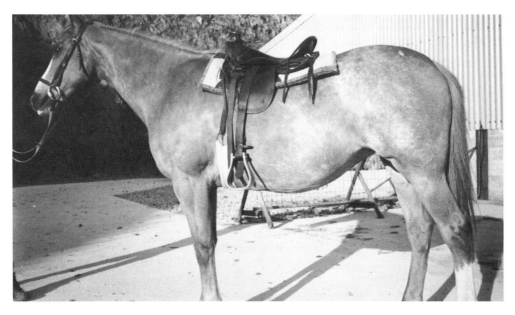

A Western saddle which keeps the seat and the leg of the rider where they should be: in the middle of the horse.

extensions were added to the hind shoes to encourage a wider stance behind and relieve the pressure on the medial surface of the hock joints. The muscles of the injured forelimb had wasted, so that as the mobility in the carpal joint increased owing to the ultrasound treatment, the range of movement had to be maintained by building up the muscle power. Weight training was introduced, using a tendon boot which was adapted with pockets for individual weights. The mare started a programme of in-hand walking exercise – usually down to the pub and back – increasing the weights and walking time over a period of six to eight weeks.

It would have been possible to treat the inflammation of the dorsal spinous processes locally, using physiotherapy. However, it was felt that the long development of compensation had affected the whole diagonal build of the horse. It was therefore better to try to redress the balance of the whole spine. This was done by a chiropractor from the McTimoney School where special training is given in animal manipulation. The chiropractor made an assessment of the saddle based on the shape and symmetry of the horse after the manipulation was carried out. The width fitting was no longer correct, so a saddler was asked to supply a saddle that met the recommendations of the chiropractor and took into account the clinical diagnosis of the referral centre. Eventually a final check of the saddle was made using computer analysis. This gave some valuable information about the way in which both riders had shifted their weight to one side and were, in fact, overloading the injured fore-limb. This seemed to be a result of their being tipped forwards by the developing stiffness of the opposite hind leg. Eventually the horse was moved to a livery yard where the working surface was kept in excellent condition, never getting too heavy or slippery, so that the mare was able to return to full ridden work in comfort.

The second case history concerns a 16hh sixteen-year old Thoroughbred gelding, who seemed to be such a powerfully built horse that, after a career as a hunter, he went to work in a riding school as a weight carrier. Although he had large shoulders and a deep girth, nobody ever really looked at his topline. They would have seen that his withers ended about six inches from his loins. Any rider of any size could not help but sit on the unsupported part of his back, over the lumbar vertebrae. He, too, went for complete diagnosis and he, too, came back with a shopping list of changes. There was navicular disease in both forefeet, inflammation of the dorsal spinous processes, pelvic tilt, spavin in both hocks, and an old stifle injury, which was probably in the form of a damaged cruciate ligament. The present owner had acquired him when the riding school closed, and had given him a caring, stress-free home. Unfortunately he was not the sort of horse that could be retired from work altogether, because he just got bored and did not know what to do with his own strength.

The major problem in keeping him in work was the fact that he could not keep shoes on. Years of concussion to the feet, and the presence of chronic white-line disease, resulted in the shoes just dropping off him after only two to three weeks.

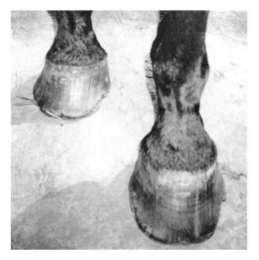

After years of wearing shoes that fell off every two weeks, this horse retired to light hacking, barefoot. The feet are not very beautiful to look at but they actually became tougher than they had been when the horse was shod.

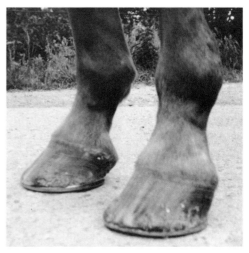

Feet that once suffered from severe laminitis: the poor quality of the horn is made up for by the quality of the shoeing.

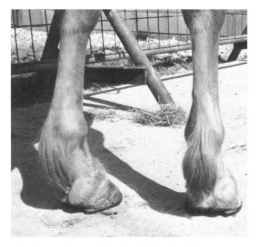

Conformation of the forelimbs in this older horse led to recurrent lameness. The generous support given to the heels by the shoes allowed the horse once more to enjoy hacking out.

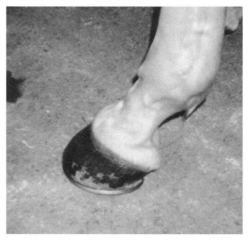

A small hoof with crumbling walls. The shoe gives the forelimb the bearing surface that really should be provided by the foot.

Extensive and persistent use of all the recommended supplements made no difference. It was considered that anything, even if it was glued on, which came into contact with the white line simply made for a more inviting medium for germs, especially in wet or muddy conditions. The other consideration was the state of the back muscles. Parts of these were in spasm, parts had no tone at all. If the back could not be made supple, the concussion on the limbs would eventually make any form of exercise intolerable.

The shoes were removed and a location was found where the horse could go barefoot in reasonable comfort. The back and hind limbs were treated firstly by chiropractic manipulation, then by acupuncture. The inevitable periods of lameness, which followed as the horse began to loosen up and resume a small amount of exercise on the lunge, were treated homoeopathically. Regular doses of high-potency *Silica* were given, together with a broad-spectrum vitamin and mineral supplement, to harden the feet. A saddle was made for him which transferred the weight of the rider to an extended bearing surface which used the support of the long back muscles and the upper surface of the ribcage, rather than lodging itself into hollows behind the withers. Constant attention was paid to the rhythm of each gait so that, as far as possible, the horse could keep himself balanced without increasing the stress to one joint or limb. The rhythm became so consistent that he was eventually able to perform light duties as a schoolmaster for his owner who wanted some lunge lessons.

The Feet

The ridden horse is locked between the saddle – with the rider in it – and the shoes attached to his feet. Considerable stress is therefore placed on the feet, which is exacerbated by ill-fitting shoes. Conversely, remedial farriery has a very important part to play in relieving many limb and foot conditions.

Of course, it is unlikely that the changes – the wear and tear – in the horse's joints and skeleton can be reversed. It is all structural damage which would require complete remodelling to return to normal. On a small scale, healing of bones, joints and ligaments is a possibility, using, for example, homoeopathy. Nevertheless, when such a considerable amount of the musculo-skeletal system has been affected, it would take more energy than is conceivable from an outside source to put it right. What can be done is to keep the muscles as supple and responsive as possible, since the pain of the joints is made worse by tightening their muscular support. An additional benefit of going barefoot is that the horse can place his feet according to how his joints feel. The position is not prescribed by the shape of the shoe. This horse seems to have adapted well to his new lifestyle; he moves fluently with a swinging back, apparently in no discomfort, thanks to the combined effects of alternative therapies.

These cases illustrate how a team approach can be used in the process of locomotor rehabilitation. In the first example, the team consisted of the clinic, a physiotherapist, a farrier, a chiropractor, a saddler and a vet. In the second example, the team consisted of the therapies themselves; chiropractic, acupuncture and homoeopathy, the clinic and the farrier. In both instances, the choice of therapies was made a great deal easier because the team was working with an accurate and comprehensive diagnosis.

COMBINING THERAPIES

Enthusiasts of one alternative medicine or another have been heard to argue that the combined use of different therapies is ill-advised because it is not possible to say which one really worked. It is probably better to assume that they all 'work', because they will all have some impact on the body's energy. They may not all have the desired effect. The diagnosis may be incorrect, or the level of energy needed to bring about a change may be simply more than is being given.

The principle of using a combination of alternative therapies is based on the idea of communication. For example, in the case of a chronic lameness, the area of tissue damage will not have an efficiently flowing blood supply. The site will be littered with damaged cells and waste products, debris which needs to be removed before any healing can take place. The use of anti-inflammatory, pain-relieving drugs is justified in the sense that, without much pain, there is a bit more mobility and the circulation can get going through areas where there has been a reduction in swelling. However, this is a bit like sending the police to a pile-up on the motorway, and forgetting to send the ambulance. The traffic gets organized, but the crash victims have to sort themselves out.

Healing means tissue repair. It means collecting the necessary materials and putting them together. This requires energy. Naturally the body has the potential to carry out its own repairs, and it is faced with the same problem of organizing its own materials to an area where the prime means of transport, via the blood stream, has broken down. In such circumstances, the body must have other means of communicating with the damaged area, otherwise it would never be able to reconstruct its own tissue. The body would begin to look like an abandoned building site, which – at least in most cases – it doesn't. Communication takes place through the electrical impulses of nerve signals, and the chemical attraction of transmitter substances. There may be pathways of energy which do not follow any solid anatomical structures. The body is able to make repairs, but that is not to say that it cannot make a better job of these repairs given a little outside help.

The object of combining alternative therapies is to get the right sort of energy to the right place at the most appropriate time. It does not do any therapy justice if it is used in a haphazard or casual way. The principles of combining the different forms of energy medicine are rather similar to those of building a railway:

1. **Carry out a complete survey**.
This may be in the form of an orthodox

veterinary investigation, using laboratory facilities, X-rays and other methods of tissue analysis, or the diagnosis may be made in terms of a particular therapy, acupuncture or homoeopathy.

2. Clear the route.

Take the most obvious limiting factor and try to eliminate it. For example, in the first case history, the limiting factor was the damage to the carpal joint. Without restoring the function here, any attempt to help the rest of the horse would have been pointless. In the case of the gelding, the shoes imposed limitations because they kept falling off. The horse was continually having to cope with a sore foot which had cast a shoe, as well as joints in any of the other limbs which were painful from having to compensate. Not wearing shoes at all, at the very least, allowed the horse's joints to find their own range of movement.

3. Lay the track.

Once the major obstacles have been removed – and this may even require some form of surgery – it is then necessary to get below all the layers of compensation. The spine is the central axis, and the nerves from the spinal cord go to all parts of the body. A smooth, uninterrupted flow of information from these nerves is the very minimum requirement before introducing forms of energy with more specific targets in mind. Chiropractic and osteopathy are both suitable means of smoothing the way. The balance of the spine also depends on the balance of the shoes. The skill of the farrier plays a large part in re-aligning the horse, and maintaining the effect of manipulation.

4. Bring on the rolling stock.

Treatment by acupuncture uses energy channels which have been mapped out over thousands of years. Acupuncture is capable of smoothing its own way and of overcoming energy blocks by itself. However in practical terms, the horse often responds so well to manipulation that further treatment is sometimes superfluous. If, on the other hand, just building the railway is not enough, then following manipulation with acupuncture to open up the flow of healing energy is appropriate.

5. The freight.

Homoeopathic remedies carry an energy imprint of their original substance. The remedy has to match a specific tissue, a special collection of symptoms or a special mental configuration. Like acupuncture, homoeopathic remedies can find their own way round the body. Nevertheless it does seem that if the energy flow in the body has already been stimulated by manipulation, or by acupuncture/acupressure, the receptivity of the tissue for homoeopathy is increased: the potency of the homoeopathic substance is itself potentized. In other words acupuncture, like goods trucks, can be used to carry homoeopathy.

All forms of medicine follow the same plan of treatment. Whatever kind of medicine is used, there has to be a diagnosis, a basis for understanding what you are about to treat. Diagnosis does not only consist of identifying the relevant disorder. It requires a substantial knowledge of what *order* looks like. This may have been gained through the study of anatomy or physiology; it may be the understanding of the concept of energy lines, or it may be something as intangible as intuition. It is diagnosis which guides the surgeon's knife, the acupuncturist's needle and the healer's hands.

A surgeon knows that diseased tissue will not heal. This has to be removed before healing can take place. The orthodox medical practitioner knows that medicines are of little use to a patient in a state of shock. All efforts are directed towards restoring the vital functions before any therapy can begin. The procedure in all forms of medicine is the same: first make the survey, then remove obstructions, then open the route for the therapy.

Where alternative medicine is different, and particularly when several therapies are used in combination, is that the routes are not prescribed. They can be directed entirely to suit the individual landscape. This is the key to their success, but the difficulty is that one is very often spoilt for choice.

When you discuss your horse's problems with other horse owners, you will often hear somebody say that they knew somebody else who had a horse 'just like that'. Well, no they didn't! They may have had a horse with the same symptoms but it is unlikely that the horses experienced them in the same way, and if they did then it is almost inevitable that the symptoms were in some way modified by the owners, or the environment. For example, an abscess in the foot can cause such severe lameness in one horse that one suspects he has broken his leg. Yet another horse tolerates the same condition, so that when, weeks later, a sliver of flint is removed from very close to the pedal bone, it is incomprehensible that the horse was not hopping about on three legs. To this we have to add the fact that one owner may poultice an abscess, one may call the farrier immediately, one may get the vet in and another may simply let nature take its course.

Each horse, his life-style, his human partner, make up an individual unit. Alternative medicine respects this individuality. That is why alternative therapies are so unsuited to scientific analysis. To quantify a system of treatment in scientific terms, you have to have identical models, with identical symptoms, receiving identical doses. This may be possible with specially bred white mice, artificially induced symptoms and laboratory conditions. Yet think of any livery yard, of its horses and their owners, of the different demands on the horse, of the different expectations of the riders. Each partnership is unique, and so are its problems.

Treatment by alternative medicine is based not on scientific evaluation but on clinical observation. The more recent developments in alternative medicine, like osteopathy, chiropractic or radionics, look back to some of the ancient medical philosophies. Therefore, in the whole spectrum of alternative medicine there are clinical observations which stretch back thousands of years. It is likely that somewhere in all that time the symptoms of one individual will have occurred before, and a solution found. There are no standardized doses in energy medicine, so there can be no prescriptions in the modern sense. However, based on the principles outlined above, the following is a guide to suggest combinations of therapies that might be used to treat specific conditions.

Diagnosis: Navicular Disease

Obstacles to clear Look at the length of stride from the shoulder downwards. Adjust the saddle width if necessary.

Smooth the energy path Progressive pain in the front feet causes the back to tighten. Loosen and rebalance the muscles of the topline by manipulation.

Create an energy carrier Remedial shoeing. This cannot have real benefit if the horse continues to take short, choppy strides. Loosen cumulative muscle tension, for example by massage and stretching exercises.

Apply specific energy When there is adequate support for the heels of the forefeet then homoeopathic treatment can be used to restore the circulation.

Diagnosis: Inflammation of the Dorsal Spinous Processes

Obstacles to clear Relieve pain around the dorsal spinous processes using physiotherapy, acupuncture or, if necessary, surgery.

Smooth the energy path Restore confidence in the use of the long back muscles by relieving spasm, or re-establishing muscle tone. Acupuncture or hands-on healing is beneficial.

Create an energy carrier Support the rehabilitation of the back, as it comes into the work, with homoeopathic remedies.

Apply specific energy Retrain and rebuild the muscular support for the spine, by long-reining and, later, lunging.

Diagnosis: Sacro-iliac strain with no fracture

Obstacle to clear Reduce the degree of pelvic tilt by chiropractic or osteopathy.

Smooth the energy path Relieve the muscle spasm which accumulates around the lumbar spine and the neck using chiropractic or acupuncture.

Create an energy carrier Maintain the process of healing when exercise is introduced by using homoeopathic remedies.

Apply specific energy Begin retraining the weaker limb using weights, or rebuild muscle wastage using electrical muscle stimulation. Protect weak tissue with homoeopathic remedies.

Diagnosis: Arthritis

(This is really a blanket diagnosis for any form of degenerative joint disease.)

Obstacles to clear Adjust the bearing surface of the shoes and the saddle to allow the horse the maximum freedom of movement.

Smooth the energy path As joints become painful, muscles tighten, and joint movement becomes even more restricted. Relieve the pain using acupuncture and homoeopathy in combination.

Create an energy carrier Make regular use of suppling exercises before and after ridden work.

Apply specific energy Homoeopathic 'arthritis' remedies, herbal supplements or healing. There are even specially formulated diets for the changing metabolism of the older horse.

Diagnosis: Unthriftiness

Obstacles to clear Check teeth, worm adequately, test blood for organ disorders, monitor heart and respiration rates.

Smooth the energy path Stimulate the flow of regenerative energy using acupuncture.

Create an energy carrier Look at dietary maintenance. Remove any possibility of intimidation from other horses. Consider using vitamin and mineral supplements.

Apply specific energy Direct homeopathic remedies to alleviate organic causes of weight loss or mental anxieties: a possible application here for Bach Flower Remedies.

Diagnosis: Respiratory Allergy

Obstacles to clear Identify the source of allergens as far as possible. This is likely to involve looking at the environment in a wider sense, stable management procedures throughout the whole yard, vegetation in the surrounding fields and exhaust fumes in built-up areas.

Smooth the energy path Some apparent allergies, like sinusitis, are actually caused by restrictions elsewhere in the body. Chiropractic is most useful to eliminate this possibility.

Create an energy carrier Stimulate the body into rethinking its response to allergens. Use stimulation of the acupuncture point for allergy.

Apply specific energy Homoeopathy or healing.

It would be almost impossible to provide an exhaustive list of conditions in the horse – at least within one volume – which could be treated according to this scheme. Every disease and disability has its own nuances which might alter the order in which the different therapies are used, or even the choice of therapies altogether. The above selection is a guide, not a gospel. The point is that every alternative therapy has a special advantage which determines when it is most appropriate for use. The order in which they follow on from one another is entirely logical; it is not a hit-or-miss approach.

There is, at present, a movement towards 'D.I.Y. medicine'. There is an increase in the availability of textbooks on physiotherapy, homoeopathy, acupressure, and herbal remedies, and there is a willingness on the part of many practitioners to share their experiences in an atmosphere of increased awareness in the horse-owning public. The most obvious motivation for taking treatment into one's own hands is the fear of incurring large vet's bills. Yet many horse owners spend a lot of money in their quest for finding their own form of treatment, before having to spend the same all over again when the vet is finally called in. There is, however, another reason for the increased interest in self-help remedies, and that is that they offer the individual the sense of doing, the feeling of being involved.

Veterinary medicine, at its present level of development, is still very much concerned with diagnosis. Technology has given us the ability to look at the body at cellular level, even to look inside the cells, at the genetic material. The therapeutic possibilities have not kept pace. Sometimes they are rather primitive by comparison. It is rather like astronomy gathering evidence of the existence of stars that are millions of miles away. We have some understanding that they contribute to our universe, but we also know that we may never go to visit them. A scientific investigation of a horse with a lameness problem, for example, may seem particularly fussy if we suspect that all we are going to come out with is a diagnostic set of labels. Better to go straight for a treatment, a herb, a homoeopathic remedy, an active attempt to solve the problem, rather than just describe it.

There is basically only one thing wrong with this method of approach. All forms of medicine have taken hundreds, if not thousands, of years to evolve. What appears on the printed page of any reference book is always a distillation of the clinical observations and experimentation that has been going on for centuries. Those practitioners who are specially trained in the skill of using one type of therapy have received a concentrated form of this knowledge.

Take, for example, the treatment of a swelling on the lower limb of the horse. Is it soft, is it fluctuating, is it hard? Is it in the skin, or under the skin? Is it a sting, or a bruise, the result of a knock, a sprain, or might it contain a tiny chip of bone? The vet with a knowledge of tissue types at the site can estimate what structure is involved. The acupuncturist with a

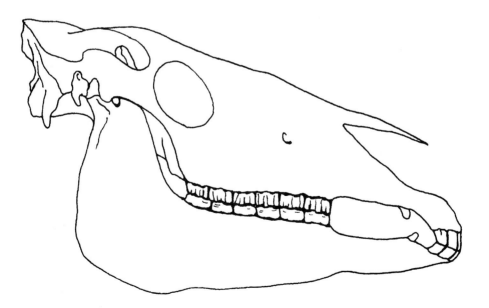

The skull of the horse showing the position of the teeth.

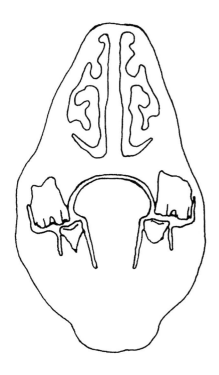

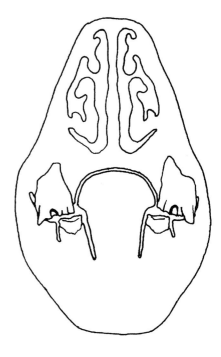

A cross-section of the skull showing the convoluted nasal passages at the top and the oral cavity below: there is very little room between the large upper molars and the cheeks.

As the back teeth grow, the outer edge begins to catch on the inside of the gums.

knowledge of energy channels can relieve the swelling by stimulating a specific acupuncture point. The physiotherapist can choose the most appropriate form of energy, perhaps laser or ultrasound, and apply it through a man-made machine. The homoeopath can select a remedy, and its potency based on the case history and/or the tissue symptoms: *Apis Mel* for oedema, *Silica* for a foreign body, *Ruta Gravis* for a splint, *Arnica* for bruising. It

will probably have taken all these professionals in excess of five years to learn their craft. There are no short cuts to understanding these practices, and likewise there should be no short cuts to treating horses either.

Most horse owners, at some time, will probably use the services of a vet, a farrier, an equine dentist, a saddler, a physiotherapist, one or more back-persons, several instructors, perhaps a mobile X-ray unit,

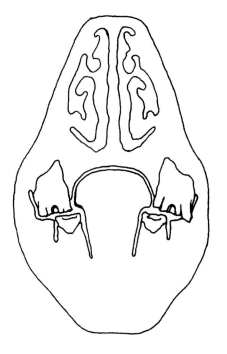

If one side of the mouth is particularly affected, this usually points to tension in the jaw, caused by musculo-skeletal problems, which can be as far away as the quarters.

a qualified nutritionist, not to mention their own back-people, the osteopath, the chiropractor, or the Alexander Technique instructor. In this line-up it is possible to collect a century's worth of expertise. Yet it doesn't count for much if they don't communicate with each other. Treatment can only be called holistic if they work together as a team.

Establishing a Team

Often enough it is the veterinary surgeon who co-ordinates the team, but there is no real reason why horse owners should not take the initiative. It's rather like being the manager of a football club: you don't have to be able to score or save a goal yourself, it's enough to know that the members of the team are in place where and when you need them.

Here is a scheme for establishing the right team for your horse:
1. The 'captain' of the team will probably be the vet, since in most countries the vet is legally responsible for the care of the horse.
2. If you wish alternative medicine to be used, is your vet sympathetic to this? Does he practise homoeopathy or acupuncture himself? If not, is he willing to refer your horse for alternative treatment to another practitioner?
3. The farrier will (it is hoped) visit your horse more regularly than your veterinary surgeon. Farriers often have to shoe horses that are not attended by the owner. If you cannot be present when
your horse is shod, follow the visit up.

Don't wait to be told if there is a problem with the shoes. Ask! Uneven wear or slight discomfort in shoeing may only indicate a minor problem now, but it might become a source of major investigation later.
4. Make sure the vet is informed of any diagnostic or remedial work carried out by the farrier. Problems suspected in the feet, like abscesses and corns, are

continued overleaf

Establishing a Team (contd.)

best dealt with by the farrier. When it comes to rebalancing the feet or remedial shoeing, it should not be forgotten that there is the rest of the horse to consider, too.

5. If you think that your horse has a back problem, or want to use back manipulation as a routine form of health care, make sure the therapist is aware of any veterinary treatment or diagnosis, even if it seems wildly improbable that there could be any interaction. Inform your vet of your intention. Let the vet and the back-person decide whether or not manipulation could be harmful.

6. Ask the equine dentist to report any uneven wear on the teeth. Tension, muscle strain, or ligament damage anywhere in the whole body can cause the horse to set his jaw and perhaps even grind his teeth. Uneven wear may indicate pain from another source or require a change in dietary management.

7. If you decide to change your saddle, be clear what it is you want to achieve by making the change. Does the saddle fit the horse? Does the saddle fit you? Does it allow you to ride as you want to, or sit as you are instructed to? Does the horse experience any difficulties, for example, going up or down hill, which might be associated with the saddle fit?

8. Makers of saddles are Masters, that is Master Craftsmen; not necessarily masters in saddle fitting. Fitting a saddle correctly is still largely based on the experience of the individual saddle-maker or retailer. Ask someone who understands the way in which the horse's back works, and who can objectively observe the horse moving under saddle, to be present at the fitting. It might be an instructor, a physiotherapist, a chiropractor or the vet. Employing an extra pair of eyes has to be money well spent for the comfort of the horse and, of course, the rider.

9. Few horses have access to extensive grazing, so there is an increased emphasis on the responsibility of the feed merchants to supply specially formulated diets. Problems like recurrent laminitis and azoturia are not uncommon, and their treatment often depends on dietary management. Many feed manufacturers have qualified nutritionists on their staff. Not only do they help formulate the feed, but they are ready to give advice and help on good feeding practice or make suggestions where there are problems. Everybody who deals with your horse professionally should be informed of his diet. This saves a conflict of advice, particularly on the feeding of supplements, where vitamins or minerals are often duplicated unnecessarily.

10. Alternative therapies continue to hold their place in competition with orthodox medicine, because they provide solutions. This would not have been possible if some specially gifted individuals had not asked a lot of questions, questions about their established professions, questions from other disciplines such as engineering, questions about the body itself. To ask questions is already to start looking for an answer. So ask questions of every practitioner who visits your horse: it furthers not only your own understanding, but also theirs.

SUMMARY

1. An holistic approach to treating the horse must involve a team effort. Having separate individuals treat different parts of the horse, though these might add up to the whole, is not the same thing at all.

2. Holistic treatment includes therapies which are not thought of as alternative: saddle fitting, dental care, and farriery.

3. There are an increasing number of groups of like-minded practitioners who now offer the team approach. They usually consist of a vet, a farrier, a professional trained to examine and treat backs, and a saddler.

4. Much of the demand for alternative medicine will be for the treatment of locomotor problems, for the simple reason that these play such a large part in orthodox veterinary practice.

5. There is no reason why alternative medicine should not be used routinely for all sorts of equine disorders. However, most equine illnesses will be attended by a veterinary surgeon who is trained first and foremost in orthodox medicine. Most acute problems respond quickly and reliably to modern medicines, and emergencies are certainly no occasion for experimentation.

6. Like any form of medical training, practitioners of alternative medicines have specialized knowledge and skills. Information is readily available on the purpose and technique of all the major therapies, in the form of handbooks. It is worth reading up about a treatment before booking the therapist.

7. Every alternative therapy aims to treat the whole individual. In an holistic approach, the treatments will overlap. Make sure that everybody involved in treating your horse communicates – with you and with each other.

8. Each form of therapy has its strong point. Sometimes the effect of therapies used in combination is more powerful than individual therapies used on their own.

9. To use an holistic approach it is necessary to visualize the whole. Of course it's possible to have a broken leg and a bad dose of flu at the same time, but often there will be a common denominator, even if the symptoms are at opposite ends of the body. The purpose of holistic medicine is to pick up the common thread and unravel it.

10. Any form of treatment must be based on diagnosis.

7

THE HEALING ART

OF RIDING

There is no secret so close as that
between a rider and his horse.
Robert Smith Surtees, *Mr Sponge's*
Sporting Tour

It is not disrespectful to suggest that the
reason we need therapies for our horses at
all is that we ride them. We don't all have
the luxury of a tundra in our backyard, any
more than we might have a prairie to ride
across. For those who live in rural areas,
there may be good access to open countryside, but in some parts of industrial Europe
most riding is confined to an indoor school
and a few designated tracks. A great many
horses live in cities and they hack out in
the company of double-decker buses. The
fact is, whatever technological wizardry
comes our way, man continues to be drawn
to the horse. Horses are kept, mostly, to be
ridden. The shape of that back just
demands to be sat on. If necessary they are
kept on pocket-handkerchief-sized pieces
of land. The horse is amazingly adaptable,
considering the variety of habitats he is

offered. Of course everybody knows of
horses whose lives have been made
unpleasant or unbearable by unsympa-
thetic riding. Yet many more horses actually thrive on their association with man
and their work under saddle.

If the perfect horse exists, most of us
probably couldn't afford him. In most
instances a horse will be purchased
because his physical build makes him suitable for the demands of a particular equestrian discipline. Some horses, however,
will be taken on as a challenge, and others
will quite simply be rescued. Whatever the
intention, the acquisition is only the starting point, the rest is down to training.

The object of riding is to achieve perfect
harmony and balance with the horse. That
is already fairly ambitious. To maintain
the balance and harmony with the horse at
speed, or going over jumps, or performing
elaborate step sequences is a very tall
order indeed. It really isn't disrespectful to
either the rider or the horse to suggest that

things are going to go wrong, and that problems will occur.

Apart from the farmer who sits on his pig to find out whether or not she is ready for mating, there is no form of communication between man and beast which relies to such a large extent on physical contact, as that between a rider and his horse. Riding is akin to playing a musical instrument, and a stringed one at that. The resonance of a stringed instrument depends very much on how it is played. In the right hands the cheapest fiddle can sound like a concert violin; in the wrong hands a Stradivarius will sound like any old lump of wood. A violin played just a little out of tune loses its roundness of tone, but this quickly returns once the tuning is spot on. The wood that goes to make the musical instrument has its own quality of resonance. This does not become vulnerable until it is actually played upon.

The horse in his natural habitat lives more or less in harmony with his own energy. There are relatively few influences which upset or overpower this balance. Of course, horses in the wild catch colds and coughs, they carry worm burdens, they injure themselves and they get stiff with old age. However, though it probably can't be statistically proven, they are not prone to navicular disease, bone spavin, bad backs, crumbly feet, or have allergies or azoturia, in fact all those disorders which, it has to be said, are unfortunately the mainstay of modern veterinary practice. A free-roaming herd of horses moves in tune with its environment, in tune with the seasons, in tune with danger, if it must. The purpose of using alternative medicine in horses is to restore this natural sense of intonation, at least as much as possible. However, where riding is concerned, it's not only the horse we are dealing with. It's not enough just to keep on fixing the instrument, if the player continues to be a little off key.

Every being has an energy field. It does not matter whether you think of this as the sum total of chemical and physical processes which differentiate living tissue from a piece of clay, or whether you can visualize the layers of subtle energy which suffuse and extend beyond the physical appearance of the body. The fact is that the horse has one energy, and a human being has another. Their metabolism is different, their biological rhythm is different, their intelligence is different. In riding, these two energies come into contact. The harmony between the horse and rider depends on whether these energies can move in sympathy, or whether they remain separate, like layers of oil on water. It therefore follows that when alternative remedies are used to restore the balance in problems associated with riding, their effect will be limited if the harmony of the horse's body is subjected to a discordant influence from the rider. On the other hand, a rider may have the skill and sensitivity to exert such a harmonizing influence over a certain type of horse that treatment by any other means becomes totally unnecessary.

The art of riding, along with its preparation, contains so many elements from each of the alternative therapies that it becomes a form of energy medicine in itself. These various elements consist of massage, manipulation, physical therapy, even acupressure and healing. The very

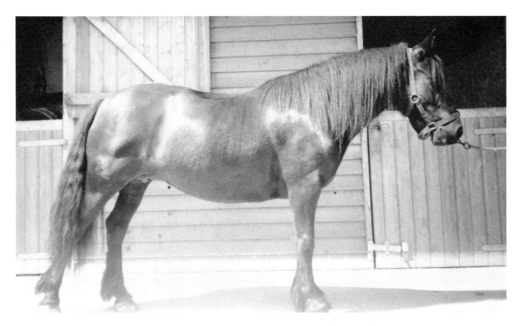

Horses are individuals, not only in size but also in shape and mentality. (Above) a Fell pony. (Below) a Dartmoor-Cross riding pony. On page 123 is an Apaloosa.

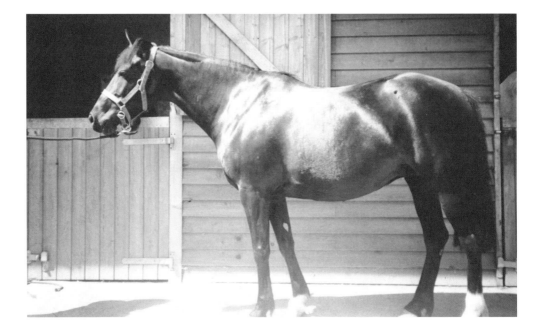

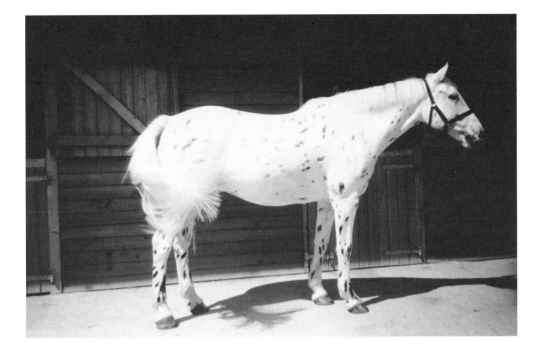

best therapy for the disorders caused by riding is, often, riding.

The art of riding begins with the horse in the stable. How does he stand? What is the height of the haynet or rack? What is the slope of the stable floor? A horse may spend twelve hours or more in the stable, especially in winter. The way in which he has to stand to reach his hay influences the way in which he is able to use his back under saddle. If the haynet is relatively high, he may have to hollow his back to reach it. Since he is likely to spend more hours in this position than he does under saddle, getting him to round his back while being ridden may meet with resistance. The same can happen when the floor slopes in the wrong direction, compared to where the horse feeds. This can be particularly

uncomfortable for horses that are themselves croup high. The dorsal spinous processes slant backwards at the withers, but forwards in the loins. In the most central part of the back they point straight up. When the back is hollowed, the dorsal spinous processes at the withers and loins press in on those in the mid-back. This causes inflammation and makes it painful for the horse to lift his back when asked by the rider. One solution is to modify the stable floor by building up the bed to even it out.

If riding begins with bringing the horse in from summer pasture, the horse's gut is often distended by the gases which form during the microbial processing of the grass in the hind gut. The tension that is caused by tightening the girth can actually create the feeling of suffocation in the horse. If the horse suddenly pulls back in panic, it can mean a visit from the chiropractor or even the vet, so it is worth letting the horse have a 'quiet' hour, without eating, before any ridden work.

PREPARING TO RIDE

Grooming is massage. It prepares the skin and the underlying tissue for contact with the tack and later the rider's weight. In addition there are some very useful stretching exercises which provide an excellent means of loosening up the horse, before you actually get into the saddle.

Grooming is a form of massage: horses are sensitive to different kinds of brush.

Stretching Exercises

FRONT LIMBS

Stretches for the front limbs are carried out before putting the saddle on, but in the same way that is used to stop the girth pinching. This helps to free the shoulders and any tightness around the withers and over the ribcage. Pull the forelimb towards you, giving the horse time to get his balance over the hindquarters. When the leg is extended, wait till the horse relaxes a little and then apply a little traction using your own body weight. If the horse is inclined to tip forward, pull the forelimb across the midline. This is a good way to alleviate any soreness which might be accumulating under the points of the saddle tree.

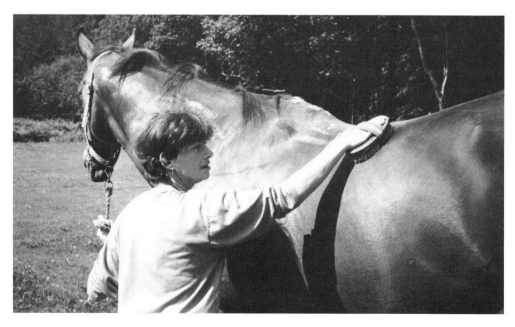

A soft body brush.

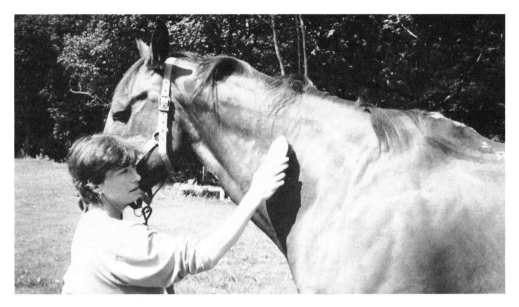

A stiff Dandy brush.

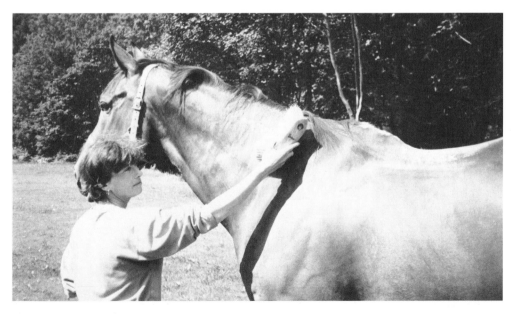

'Flicking' with a soft, long-bristled brush. This is more a form of Therapeutic Touch than grooming.

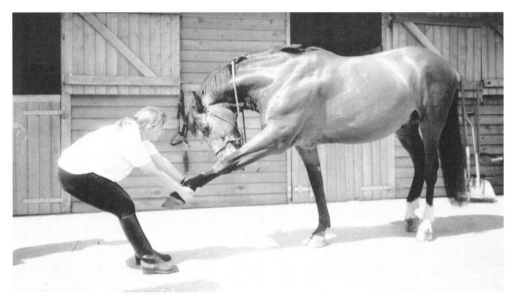

Stretching the forelimb: the benefits of this exercise extend right under the saddle area.

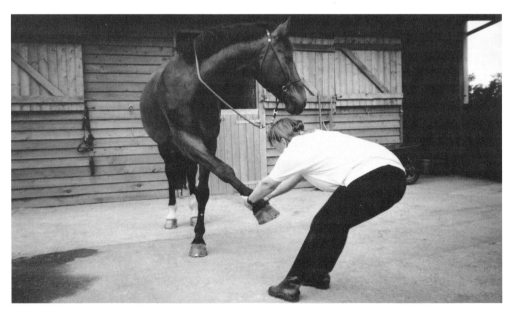

A variation of the forelimb stretch, bringing the leg across the midline: a good way of stretching areas that may have been compressed by a narrow saddle tree.

HIND LIMBS

Two or three flexions of the hind limbs are good warm-up exercises, especially for the older horse. Lift one hind leg and place just the toe forwards on to the ground under the horse's belly. Lift the leg again and bring it out to the side, letting the toe touch the ground. Lift once more and draw the leg back as far as possible, again letting only the toe touch the ground. Many horses find this last position difficult because they have tight areas of muscle in the quarters. Do not force the leg: the degree of stretch can be increased with each practice, and gives the horse confidence to use the hind limbs when working under saddle.

NECK AND BACK

Neck and back stretches are a good way of checking that the horse has not developed any muscle problem from lying awkwardly in the stable. They are a good all-round exercise both before and after ridden work. They involve using carrots, so for some horses they are best after work as a reward. Stand the horse alongside a wall, so that he cannot move his quarters away; stand by his quarters on the other side and offer him a carrot from a position level with the point of his hip. As he fixes his teeth on the carrot pull it gently towards you. This encourages the muscles of the neck to relax and increases the length bend. To repeat the exercise on the other side, don't forget to turn the horse so that again he cannot move his quarters.

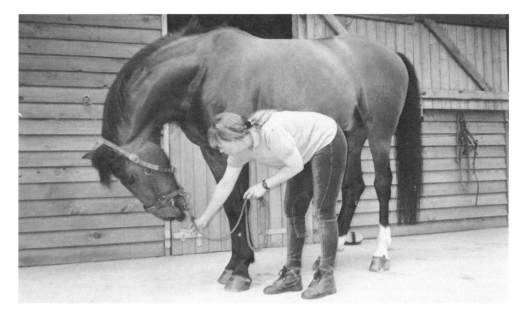

Learning to stretch the topline with a little encouragement from a carrot.

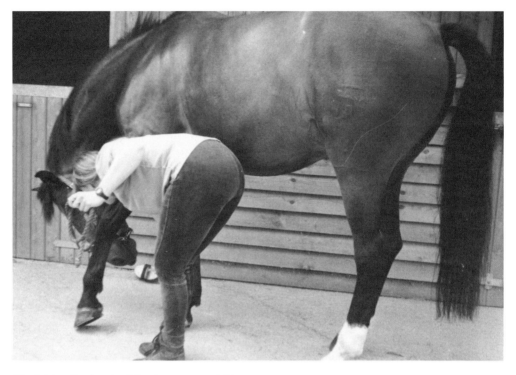

Stretching the back of the horse – and rider.

The most valuable exercise of all is the one which stretches the long back muscles, especially in the area behind the saddle. Imagine a point on the ground immediately behind the mid-point of the girth. Offer the horse a carrot from this position. It takes a little more practice but they soon get the hang of it. The less the horse spreads or drops a foreleg to get the reward, the more he will have to lift the lumbar spine, and the greater the suppling effect. This stretch can be carried out from the other end, by gently applying traction at the base of the tail. It is a useful alternative, but perhaps not quite so thorough – and of course, there's no reward for the horse.

The Saddle

Traditional Chinese medicine has given us the concept of energy lines. They appear, in all the illustrations, to run on the surface of the body. However, they actually represent channels of energy below the skin. These channels are created by the flow of electrical and nutritional energy as it makes its way around the body. Some of the channels run parallel to the spine, others run up and down the limbs. There are points along the channels next to the spine, which relate diagnostically to the limb channels. For example, if a point on the back which represents the kidney channel is painful, it means that there is a problem somewhere along that channel. The problem may be in the internal part of the channel where it enters the organ that gives it its name, or the problem may be on the outer branch of the channel somewhere along the inside of the hind limb of the horse, for instance, at the hock or stifle. If the points along the back become painful when a limb has a problem, then presumably the reverse is also true: if the points along the back have a problem, then part of a limb will become painful. Many of these diagnostic points lie directly under the saddle. If the flocking of the saddle is uneven or lumpy, the bearing surface will exert pressure on parts of these energy channels, in effect interrupting the free flow of energy along the back. The result is lameness. There is no conclusive evidence to prove it, but it often seems to be the case that the area of pain in a limb corresponds to the channel of energy which has its diagnostic point directly under the offending part of the saddle.

However, if this is the consequence of a poorly fitting saddle, then we would have to expect the opposite to happen with a well-fitting saddle. A correctly

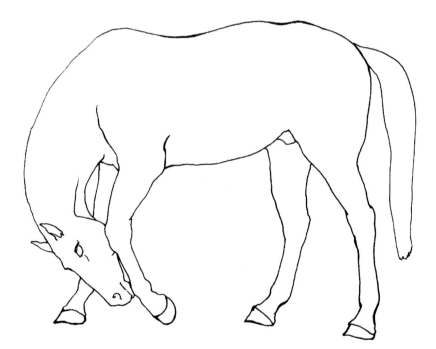

The topline is stretched as the horse reaches for a carrot that has been placed on the floor, between the forelegs and underneath the girth area. Some horses are inclined to cheat!

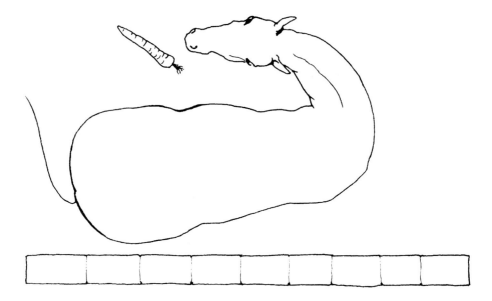

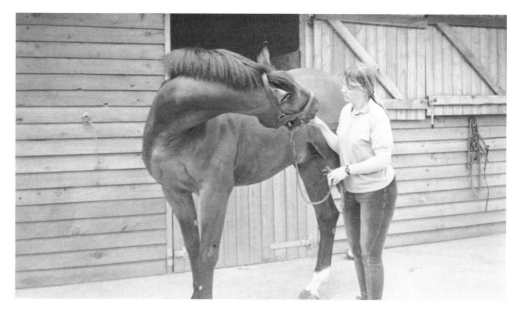

Neck stretches are best done with the horse standing parallel to the stable wall.

Neck stretching to the left.

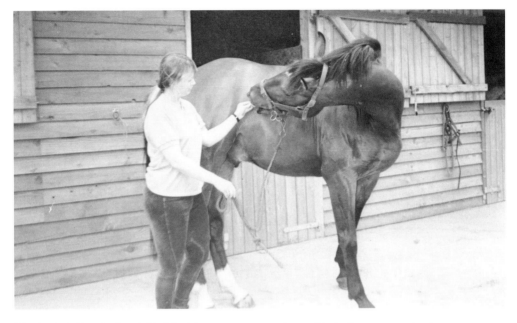

Neck stretching to the right. Most horses are accustomed to being approached from the near side, so turning this way sometimes needs a little practice.

fitting saddle with a smooth bearing surface and no pressure hotspots, must contribute to the free flow of energy, and even help to restore the fluent movement of the limbs and back. Although the horse's movement will always be slightly compromised by the mere fact of wearing a saddle at all, there is no doubt at all that a well-fitting and comfortably flocked saddle can keep these compromises to a minimum.

Stimulating the acupuncture points by light touch is the basis of acupressure. The saddle should really only be an interface between the seat of the rider and the back of the horse. If the saddle is well fitted and well balanced to both the horse and the rider, then it is the rider's seat which has the last word in the energy stakes. In other words, the way in which the rider uses his backside through the saddle can be as beneficial to the horse's well being as hands used in the art of acupressure. In many ancient cultures the flow of energy in parallel with the spine was not only of physical but also of spiritual significance. In horse riding, the human spine is vertical to the horizontal spine of the horse and the influence of the human energy is the same. What effect this has on the horse depends on the sum total of the rider's physical and emotional make-up. All this converges on the horse through the rider's seat. At its most harmonious, the influence a rider

Balanced Riding

In riding, reflexes are activated and movement sequences are practised. If the horse fails to respond to a command, we talk about him 'not understanding'. In fact, the lack of response or inaccuracy of movement depends not on the horse's understanding but on the rider's. If the rider pushes the right button then the horse can do little else but carry out the correct movement, as long as it is within his capability. A rider has it in his power to influence the movements of the horse to the extent that they can be rhythmical and in balance, or arhythmical and lop-sided. Rather than practising walk, trot and canter, it is probably more appropriate to practise rhythm. An equal footfall in four, two or three time, means an equal stride length and, if this is the case, the horse has more chance of working in balance. A well-balanced horse is less likely to suffer from injury through strain. This is riding as physical therapy.

might have over a horse comes very close indeed to healing.

When somebody once asked the way to Carnegie Hall, one of the most famous concert venues in the world, the answer he got was 'practice, practice, practice'. Well, even the most famous musicians don't always play in tune, and riders are not always able to ride in total harmony with their horses. With horses it's not just practice that makes perfect. The horse's balance can be affected by shoeing; rough edges on teeth can cause tension in the jaw; competitive riding is demanding and injuries or strains are bound to happen. Yet, whereas few riders would attempt to shoe their own horses, and not many would rasp their own horses' teeth, there is one way for the rider to restore the fine-tuning of the horse when imbalances do occur, and that is by using homoeopathy. It is not a substitute for good riding, or thorough training, but as an aid to re-establishing the harmony, it gets right under the saddle.

Using Remedies

Homoeopathic remedies are given in dilutions, which contain an imprint of the energy of the original substance. Any substance can be prepared homoeopathically, from animal, vegetable or mineral sources. Even something as insoluble as flint – which becomes homoeopathic *Silica* – can be made into a remedy. It is repeatedly ground up and mixed with lactose until the particles are so small that they can be suspended in a fluid. This can then be shaken and diluted in the prescribed homoeopathic way. The remedies relieve symptoms which they would otherwise cause if the substances were taken in their natural state. For example, a person with gastroenteritis may show symptoms that resemble acute poisoning with arsenic. This substance (in homoeopathic form) is actually used to cure the symptoms it would cause.

In order to use the remedies correctly it is necessary to know what the symptoms of each substance are, in their natural and poisonous form. There is an almost unlimited number of remedies to be had, and getting to know the drug picture of all of them, especially in the way that relates to animal treatment, takes a great deal of experience. In many cases, where serious or chronic disorders are to be treated, it will be necessary to get help from a trained homoeopath, who can translate the symptoms of the animal into the correct homoeopathic remedy.

Nevertheless, there are remedies that have a few well-defined characteristics or even a particular affinity to certain types of tissue. This makes it possible to apply them in a way similar to the way in which we are accustomed to applying orthodox medicines. One of the attractions of homoeopathy is that the remedies are specific, but this also makes for one of the difficulties in choosing the suitable substance. For example, when a horse goes lame we might put him on a short course of Bute. We suspect a bruised sole, but it could just as easily be a mild sprain or a hard knock. At any rate, the horse eventually goes sound and we are generally none the wiser. Using homoeopathy requires a bit more forethought, but the end result is rather more satisfying because it serves to confirm our diagnosis.

STARTING A COLLECTION OF REMEDIES

Many of the homoeopathic pharmacies provide 'starter' packs for home use. This is a bit like putting the cart before the horse, because it encourages us to try to fit symptoms described by the remedies we have on the shelf to those of the animal, rather than vice versa. In starting a collection of homoeopathic remedies it is perhaps better to consider what you are actually going to use them for. It has to be said in caring for a horse, that there are some occasions when expert medical attention will be required. Colic is **ALWAYS** an emergency, as are major wounds or severe bleeding. Acute laminitis, bronchial spasm, high fever and azoturia, also require professional help of one sort or another. Of course, all these conditions can be treated by alternative methods, but only by the most confident and competent practitioner. In cases such as these, the straightforward orthodox veterinary approach is likely to provide the most reliable relief in the first instance.

Homoeopathic remedies really come into their own for the rider, as a means of coping with incidents that occur while training or competing and which upset the balance of the musculo-skeletal system. In this respect they should be looked on as a form of 'working' medicine, an extra implement in the grooming kit, as necessary to the day-to-day running of the horse as a hoof-pick or a bodybrush. The most usual types of injury are going to be knocks and bangs, cuts and grazes, pulled muscles, ligaments and tendons, overreach injuries, puncture wounds, possibly with foreign bodies involved, and wrenched nerves. Bearing all this in mind, I would suggest that the following remedies would make a sensible start to the collection.

The Horse Owner's Homoeopathic Starter Kit

Arnica Regulates the blood circulation, whether it be in the form of local damage to a blood vessel, which is a bruise, or generalized disturbance of the blood circulation, which is shock.

Rhus Toxicodendron An affinity with muscles and joints. Relieves pain in cramped muscles, which allows joints to move more freely. A 'training' remedy for hard-working muscles that loosen up with exercise, but not completely. A 'must' for the older horse, where arthritic stiffness improves with movement.

Bryonia This is included because the affinity with muscle fibre and joint tissue is similar to **Rhus tox**. However, the main indication for its use is that the symptoms become worse from movement. Realistically speaking, if this is the case with a horse in work, the cause should first be thoroughly investigated before choosing this remedy.

Ruta Graveolens This remedy acts on the periosteum, the sensitive covering of the bones and on cartilage. Together with **Rhus tox**, the combination can be applied to most injuries that involve the musculoskeletal system.

Hypericum This remedy has an affinity with nerves, and can be used both for pain relief (pain being the result of irritated nerve fibres), or where a wrench or sprain might have overstretched the nerve fibres and caused damage.

Silica A remedy for connective tissue, abscesses and the elimination of foreign bodies; being flint, it is also a homoeopathic hoof hardener.

Hepar Sulf Often said to be the homoeopathic equivalent of an antibiotic. It is used in cases of infection where there is pus formation. Very low potencies promote the discharge; high potencies dry the discharge up.

Apis Mellifica This remedy is prepared from the bee and used to treat symptoms reminiscent of a bee sting, that is oedema. If there is fluid retention around the sheath, abdomen or lower chest, the involvement of such an organ as the liver or heart, maybe be indicated so this should be investigated.

Ledum Palustre A valuable remedy for puncture wounds. Where germs have been almost 'injected' beneath the skin, this remedy can be combined with **Hypericum**, especially where the risk of Tetanus infection is a consideration in unvaccinated horses.

Aconitum For sudden fright or anticipatory fear. The fright of sudden pain in an illness such as laminitis is a case for this remedy, or the fear in anticipating situations such as being left alone in the stable. Care should be exercised in using high potencies where there is the likelihood of strenuous activity. There appears to be quite a fall in blood pressure in some horses, which could lead to an undesirable lack of attention in a sporting event.

Rescue Remedy This is not strictly speaking a homoeopathic remedy, but it certainly should have a place in any first-aid box. It is made from the essence of wild flowers: Star of Bethlehem, for shock; Rock Rose, for terror and pain; Impatiens, for mental stress and tension; Cherry Plum, for desperation; Clematis, for the faraway feeling which often precedes loss of consciousness. These are all Bach Flower Remedies in their own right. Dr Edward Bach's intention was to find a means of healing through the personality. He wrote, 'Take no notice of the disease, think only of the outlook on life of the one in distress'. Since we probably cannot do this adequately in circumstances of great emergency, the combination of remedies in the Rescue Remedy should cover most eventualities for both humans and horses.

Administering Remedies

Homoeopathic remedies can be used as drops, pills or powders. The pills should not be handled more than is absolutely necessary because the substance is on the outside and reacts with the oils on the skin of the hands. Drops transferred to a needleless syringe and given into the side of the mouth ensures that the horse has had the remedy. The substances are quickly absorbed by the gums and don't have to be swallowed, but tablets can be 'packaged' in a carrot for convenience.

Strictly speaking, there is no such thing as a dose in homoeopathy. The remedy is a form of energy and therefore what is good for a hamster is also good for an elephant. In practical terms, if you want to be absolutely sure that your horse has had the necessary 'amount', use about eight of the tiny tablets for a 15hh horse, or ten to twelve drops. Given over a long period, it is possible for the remedy to invoke the very symptoms you are trying to cure. In the short term, if the remedy is not appropriate there is simply no response. Where

the specific symptoms get worse immediately, within 24 hours of giving a homoeopathic remedy, this is usually a sign that the match is particularly good and that the remission is going to be successful. *Arnica* is generally used in 6 or 30 potency, which is quite low. This is because its use is usually associated with an acute situation, and it is likely to be given several times in the course of one day. Otherwise high potencies are preferable, beginning with a potency of 200. Even as treatment for recent injuries, the metabolism of animals seems to make the higher energy status of these potencies more applicable.

Practical Homoeopathy

The best way to get acquainted with practical homoeopathy is to work with just two or three remedies. *Arnica* and Rescue Remedy are top of the list, but since *Rhus Tox* and *Ruta Gravis* have a strong affinity with the musculo-skeletal system, these have to be the mainstay of any homoeopathic treatment for 'training' injuries. Here are a few examples of incidents which might occur at any time in any yard, and for which the homoeopathic remedies proved invaluable.

A horse received a nasty kick on the inside of the hind leg, between the hock and the stifle. The tear had to be stitched and there was concern about bruising. The horse was given an antibiotic injection, and *Arnica 30* was given three time a day. Two days later the wound was checked and, though all looked well, it was decided that infection could still complicate the healing process, and a second antibiotic injection was given. A few seconds later the horse began to stagger about, showing all the signs of an allergic reaction to the injection, which had consisted of Penicillin. If the horse had gone into shock, he might well have died from the collapse of his circulation. As it was, he managed to keep himself moving, trotted in a wobbly fashion up the road, and was discovered a mile away eating from the grass verge as if nothing had happened. It can't be proved, but it is likely that the *Arnica* helped to stabilize the circulation, and probably saved his life.

A polo pony was hit badly on the side of the head during play. He suffered a severe nose bleed, but seemed otherwise undistressed. The bleeding had ceased, when all of a sudden the pony lay down on the ground, apparently out for the count. Despite the efforts of the little crowd that gathered, the pony was not to be roused. An onlooker happened to have some Arnica tablets in her handbag. These were wedged into the pony's mouth. Ten minutes later it stood up. The pony was pronounced fit to make the three-hundred mile journey home with the rest of the team, the same evening.

An aged pony belonging to a group of the Riding for the Disabled Association had been on a high dose of Bute for his arthritis. He was unable to flex any joints in the lower front limbs, and in order to pick his feet out, the forelimbs had first to be pulled forwards and then the joints flexed manually, one by one. There seemed little justification in keeping him going in such a painful state, but it was decided to have one last go to make him comfortable, this time using homoeo-

pathy. Ten days after he had started receiving regular doses of *Rhus tox*, the pony was so lively that, for a time he could not be used for teaching.

Albert was a donkey and something of a village celebrity. He had to reach his stable up a small incline, and one evening, on coming in from the field, he tripped awkwardly on the slope. He was unable to bear weight at all on his left foreleg, so that the emergency diagnosis was either a fracture of the shoulder joint or a severe dislocation. Albert was given the thumbs down. However, celebrities are not to be dispatched as easily as all that and homoeopathic help was sought. In fact the donkey had caught his toe, which was actually due for trimming, and in doing so, wrenched the whole of the forelimb. Since the injury involved all the elements of the musculo-skeletal system, *Ruta Gravis* and *Rhus Tox* were used in combination, with *Arnica* for the inevitable bruising, and three weeks later the donkey was perfectly mobile again.

A hunter mare developed a flat swelling over the ribcage, which was described as being the size of a dinner plate. The owner suspected a thorn was lodged there, though a wound was hardly visible. The size of the swelling was indeed no exaggeration. The horse was treated with Silica, and within three days the owners were able to recover the thorn, and the swelling resolved.

An aged hunter gelding caught the inside of the bulb of the heel on one hind leg. This made a large cut in the soft tissue which immediately became infected. The horse, quite understandably, went lame. Although the wound was poulticed the horse was given *Hepar Sulf* in high potency. Poulticing became completely unnecessary, as the wound simply dried up within three days, and the horse then went back to work.

These examples are not prescriptions, nor are they meant to be a substitute for good professional advice, which in most instances is likely to come from a veterinary surgeon. However, in non-emergency situations, most owners will choose to observe their animals for perhaps twenty-four hours, rather than call the vet unnecessarily. This is perfectly acceptable, but it does not mean that nothing can be done in the meantime to begin the healing process. Therefore, rather than starting with the symptoms of the remedies on the shelf, try starting at the other end – with the horse. Recall the incident which has given cause for concern. Put yourself in the place of the horse and imagine what bit of you would hurt in the same situation. Did the horse get in a muddle over a jump, did he get a pole between his legs, did he land awkwardly? Did he slip on a tarmac road? Did a car stop very close behind him causing him to jolt forwards? Was the surface of the school slippery causing him to take tense, cautious strides? Imagine what the movement felt like to the horse. In many cases the answer will be a pulled area of muscle, or a strained ligament. Nevertheless, experience in treating acute mishaps first hand is not only immensely satisfying, but also gives you the confidence to treat more chronic disorders, like the arthritic conditions of older horses, using the great variety of remedies that homoeopathy has to offer.

Volumes have been written on homoeopathy since its invention, both on the substances themselves and on their application. This gives the impression that homoeopathy is an unwieldly and intellectual form of medicine, not well suited to the speed of the present century. In fact, homoeopathy is an extremely modern form of medicine, one might almost call it 'smart medicine'. Technology has given us the smart card and the smart building, where smart means the ingenious ability of inanimate objects apparently to think for themselves. Smart cards record and exchange information, smart buildings can control their own internal climate, by opening or shutting their windows and blinds. It would seem appropriate to have a medicine that could perform in the same way. Homoeopathy matches an energy deficit with an energy pattern. If the match is not good enough, then it doesn't do anything. That's a pretty smart form of medicine.

IN CONCLUSION

'*Similia similibus curentur*': let likes be treated by likes. This philosophy was the basis for Hahnemann's development of the homoeopathic principle. In the riding horse, most of the problems we have to treat will be caused by riding. In *Alice in Wonderland*, The White Knight proclaimed, 'The great art of riding is to keep your balance properly', and promptly fell heavily on top of his head. Both in the use of alternative medicine and in the art of riding, there will also be times when we land on our feet.

SUMMARY

1. The key elements of riding are balance, suppleness and flexibility. The rider can either dominate the horse and suppress the horse's energy with his own, or unite with the horse to form a harmonious whole.

2. The intention of alternative medicine is to create harmony, both physically and mentally. Therefore riding has the power to be used as a form of healing.

3. The influence of shoeing and the saddle should not be underestimated. In riding, the horse's body is sandwiched between the two.

4. More important than training the walk, trot, or canter, is to practise rhythm. Listen carefully to the hoofbeats. If one or two are more pronounced than others the horse is not working in balance. This must cause tension and eventually strain.

5. In the older horse, where there may be symptoms of arthritis which restrict the length of stride, it is probably preferable to keep a working rhythm in time with the stiffer limb(s), rather than force the horse out of balance.

6. Homoeopathic medicine is the most useful form of alternative therapy for immediate home use.

7. If the remedy is wide of the mark it will have no effect. If it is a good match, it can quickly resolve strains and injuries to the musculo-skeletal system, which, though minor at the time, might become progressively worse in the long run.

8. Get accustomed to using a few remedies and observe their effects. Begin by deciding what it is you want to treat, and what you expect the remedy to achieve.

9. In locomotor disorders, homoeopathy is often more potent when preceded by manipulation, or acupuncture.

10. Alternative medicine is 'smart' medicine, but it's even smarter not to need it in the first place. Riders have the power to to heal: they need only look to themselves.

According to Bedouin legend, Allah created the horse from a handful of the South Wind, saying 'I have given thee the power of flight without wings'. This is why we keep horses, this is why we want to ride them. All the alternative medicine in the world cannot give us the feeling of triumph and exhilaration which comes from achieving a moment's perfect harmony with the horse. Alternative medicine is an energy aid, but the only real way to balance the energy of riding is to ride with more balance. The ancient Greeks gave us the concept of treating like with like, and from Xenophon we have this advice about riding: 'Teach your horse to go with a light hand on the bit, yet to carry his neck and bend his head, then you will make him do exactly what he himself delights in'. Whereas the White Knight said, 'Plenty of practice,' as Alice helped him to his feet, again.

POSTSCRIPT

This book has been a journey, from the outer limits of the body through the inner forces that give us life, from the heart of the rider right through to the heart of the horse.

If the reader now has the feeling that there must be many more unexplored parts of this land of alternative medicine then it was a journey worth taking. Thank you for coming with me.

GLOSSARY

Acupressure Finger pressure massage applied to specific points along the energy channels of the body, as in acupuncture. The energy has a directional flow. Massage should always be used in the correct direction.

Acupuncture According to the tradition of Chinese medicine, energy (Qi) flows around the body in channels (also called meridians). The energy is kept in balance by the complementing qualities of Yin and Yang. Energy out of balance produces symptoms of illness. This is treated by inserting needles at specific points along the channels. Manipulation of the needles can be either tonifying or sedating, depending on whether the energy is in excess or deficient.

Alexander Technique A method of teaching postural awareness. Bad posture can be caused by psychological problems. It results in the constriction of movement, stiff joints, shallow breathing, impaired circulation and backache. Overcoming postural difficulties helps to alleviate the psychological tension and, therefore, its consequences.

Aromatherapy The application of aromatic and therapeutic essential oils which contain complex molecules. They are applied either through the skin (e.g. by massage or bathing) or by inhalation. The molecules are absorbed into the bloodstream or reach the brain by stimulation of the olfactory nerves.

Autogenic Training A series of mental exercises using visualization techniques which induce relaxation.

Ayurvedic Medicine The ancient holistic healing system of India. Like Traditional Chinese Medicine, the medical philosophy is concerned with balancing energies. Treatments include medicines made from herbs, minerals and vegetables, as well as practical therapies such as massage.

Bach Flower Remedies The essence of thirty-eight plants used to restore all aspects of mental harmony in a sick person, and in this way assist self-healing.

Biochemic Tissue Salts Some disorders are thought to be caused by a lack of certain minerals in the body. The natural balance is restored by using any of twelve basic tissue salts (e.g. Phosphate of Iron or

Chloride of Soda) given in homoeopathic preparation.

Biofeedback The practice of learning to control a mental or physical condition by measuring changes in the body that can be seen, heard or felt. For example, a migraine headache can be eased by imagining the hands are cooler, which lowers the electrical resistance of the skin.

Chiropractic A biomechanical treatment involving the manipulation of joints and muscles, particularly those around the spinal column.

Colour Therapy Electromagnetic wavelengths of light include colours which are visible to the eye, and ultraviolet and infrared light, which are known to have healing properties. Colour therapists work with energy centres of the body (Chakras) which are associated with different physical and mental states and which have corresponding colours.

Crystal and Gem Healing Crystals, and precious and semi-precious stones have a resonance which is thought to correspond to different levels of vibrational energy in the body.

Dowsing A diagnostic aid used in various therapies, e.g. herbalism, homoeopathy, colour therapy and radionics.

Feldenkrais Method The practice of achieving postural awareness through movement. The physical exercises are designed to achieve efficiency of movement with the minimum effort.

Healing A way of restoring health by nonphysical means. A healer acts as a medium to channel healing energy into the body.

Herbalism Medicine using pharmaceutically active ingredients of plants as they occur in natural combination, rather than purified substances which may be less effective or have harmful side-effects.

Homoeopathy A system of preparing substances from any source – animal, vegetable or mineral – and giving infinitesimal doses of it, to treat those symptoms which would be caused by taking the substance in its natural and usually toxic state.

Hydrotherapy The use of water to cleanse and heal, to increase or restrict circulation, to invigorate or relax the soft tissues of the body or as a carrier for all manner of therapeutic substances. Water is the most versatile of all therapeutic agents.

Iridology A means of diagnosing disorders by observing the colourings and markings on the iris of the eye.

Kinesiology A means of diagnosing energy imbalances in the body by testing the response of specific muscles. It takes into account the way muscle function may be influenced by food substances. Applied Kinesiology incorporates elements of acupressure and chiropractic.

Massage Kneading or stroking the soft tissue structures of the body to increase circulation, stimulate nerve endings and improve lymphatic drainage. The associated endorphin release aids pain relief.

Osteopathy An holistic approach to treating the body by adjusting muscles and joints. The osteopathic 'lesion' refers to joints which have become fixed at the extreme limit of their normal range of movement. Relieving the strain on elements of the musculo-skeletal system eases the pressure on internal organs, helping the body to heal itself naturally. A highly specialized form of osteopathy –

cranial osteopathy – has recognized a relationship between the movements of joints in the skull (cranium) and restricted movement elsewhere in the body.

Physiotherapy This is no longer really considered an alternative form of medicine, yet it uses elements from practically all of the above. It incorporates the simplest application of heat or cold, along with sophisticated electronic means of delivering energy at scientifically calculated dose rates. In many ways it is the energy medicine of the twentieth century.

Radionics/Radiesthesia A means of detecting distortions in the energy pattern of an individual through the energy waves of a 'witness', either a lock of hair, or a drop of blood.

Reflexology Pressure and massage are applied to the soles of the feet to regulate the flow of energy within ten associated zones in the body.

Rolfing A system of deep, and often painful, massage and manipulation of muscles and connective tissue used to realign the body.

Shiatsu A modern link between Western and Oriental medicine, which uses a combination of massage on acupuncture points with elements of physiotherapy and chiropractic. Pressure is exerted using fingers, thumbs, elbows, knees and even feet. The aim is to free the flow of Qi, as well as stimulating the endorphin release, and improving the circulation and lymphatic drainage.

Therapeutic Touch A technique that seems to resemble hands-on healing, but the therapy is said to be based on the concept of quantum mechanics. The intention is to balance the energy within the patient by using the extended energy field that surrounds the patient's body.

Yoga A system of exercises that combines stretching and breathing control, with relaxation and meditation. The techniques can have a profound, beneficial effect on the metabolic rate, blood pressure and brain waves.

INDEX